WHAT TO EAT

During Cancer Treatment

WHAT TO EAT
During Cancer Treatment

100 GREAT-TASTING, FAMILY-FRIENDLY
RECIPES TO HELP YOU COPE

Jeanne Besser
Kristina Ratley, RD, CSO, LDN
Sheri Knecht, RD, CSO, CNSD, LDN
Michele Szafranski, MS, RD, CSO, LDN

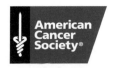

American
Cancer
Society®

Published by the
American Cancer Society
Health Promotions
250 Williams Street NW
Atlanta, GA 30303-1002

Printed in Canada

Photography: Joey Ivansco
Food Styling: Jeanne Besser
Nutritional Analysis: Madelyn Wheeler, MS, RD
Design and Composition: Jill Dible
Project Supervising Editor: Jill Russell

7 8 9   15 16 17

Library of Congress Cataloging-in-Publication Data

What to eat during cancer treatment : 100 great-tasting, family-friendly recipes to help you cope / Jeanne Besser ... [et al.].
p. cm.
Includes index.
ISBN-13: 978-1-60443-005-9 (pbk. : alk. paper)
ISBN-10: 1-60443-005-2 (pbk. : alk. paper)
1. Cancer—Diet therapy—Recipes. I. Besser, Jeanne.
RC271.D52W53 2009
641.5'631—dc22
                                  2009019771

AMERICAN CANCER SOCIETY
Managing Director, Content: Chuck Westbrook
Director, Book Publishing: Len Boswell
Managing Editor, Books: Rebecca Teaff, MA
Books Editor: Jill Russell
Book Publishing Coordinator: Vanika Jordan, MSPub
Editorial Assistant, Books: Amy Rovere

For more information about cancer, contact your American Cancer Society at **800-227-2345** or **cancer.org**.

Quantity discounts on bulk purchases of this book are available. Book excerpts can also be created to fit specific needs. For information, please contact the American Cancer Society, Health Promotions Publishing, 250 Williams Street NW, Atlanta, GA 30303-1002, or send an e-mail to **trade.sales@cancer.org**.

Table of Contents

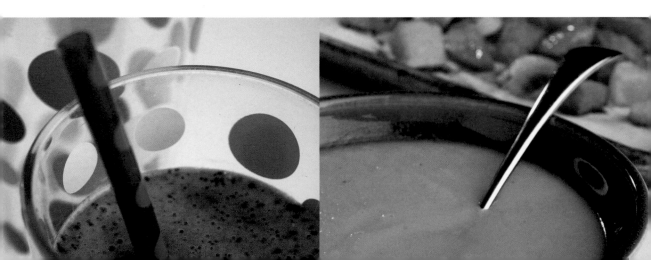

Note to the Reader

Throughout this book, you will see these icons:

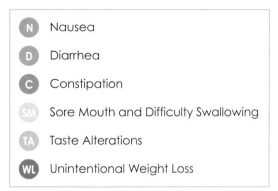

N   Nausea

D   Diarrhea

C   Constipation

SM   Sore Mouth and Difficulty Swallowing

TA   Taste Alterations

WL   Unintentional Weight Loss

The recipes in this book are organized according to symptoms: nausea, diarrhea, constipation, sore mouth and difficulty swallowing, taste alterations, and unintentional weight loss. However, many of the recipes in the book are appropriate for more than one side effect. When you see the icon for one of the symptoms listed above (either alongside the recipe or in the list of recipes on the next few pages), it means that the recipe is also appropriate for that side effect.

The nutrition information shown for each recipe represents one serving. Optional ingredients and ingredients listed without measurement (such as salt and pepper) are not represented in the analysis. When two choices are given, the first was used in the analysis.

The information in this book is not official policy of the Society and is not intended as medical advice to replace the expertise and judgment of your cancer care team. It is intended to help you and your family make informed decisions, together with your doctor.

Your doctor may have reasons for suggesting a treatment plan different from the suggestions in this book. Don't hesitate to ask him or her questions about your treatment options.

For more information about cancer and cancer treatment,
contact the American Cancer Society at 800-227-2345
or visit our Web site at cancer.org.

Recipe List by Symptom

Chapter 3. Constipation

Chapter 4. Sore Mouth and Difficulty Swallowing

Chapter 5. Taste Alterations

Chapter 6. Unintentional Weight Loss

Introduction

If you are reading this, you or someone you know is probably going through—or preparing to go through—cancer treatment. This can be a stressful and difficult time, a time filled with challenges and change.

No one can predict how cancer treatment will affect you. Not everyone experiences side effects and, for those who do, not everyone has the same side effects or reacts to treatment in the same way. Some people going through cancer treatment continue to enjoy eating and have a normal appetite throughout treatment. Others have days when they don't feel like eating at all. For many, side effects come and go.

People with cancer have unique nutritional needs and issues related to eating; what's more, these needs may change throughout the cancer experience. Your appetite may change from day to day. Foods may not taste or smell the way they did before treatment. You may be surprised by some of the foods that appeal to you during your treatment. Cancer and cancer treatments can also cause nausea, vomiting, diarrhea, constipation, mouth sores, and swallowing problems, all of which affect what and how you eat. You may have to deal with weight loss or weight gain. Weight loss can lead to weakness and fatigue.

No matter what side effects you may experience, nutrition is an essential part of dealing with cancer and cancer treatment. During your treatment, you will be concentrating on fighting cancer. Eating well will help keep you strong and supply you with the nutrients your body needs. Maintaining good nutrition will help you feel better and stay stronger.

Eating as well as you can during your treatment and your recovery is an important part of taking care of yourself. There are no hard and fast rules about how to eat during cancer treatment. Eat as healthfully as possible—the importance of this cannot be overstated. However, do not be too hard on yourself if you have days on which your appetite is poor. In some of the recipes, we list ingredients you can include to add more calories and flavor, depending on how you are feeling. Some of these ingredients are not necessarily things we would encourage as a regular part of your daily diet, such as using full-fat dairy products to increase calories or ingredients high in sodium to add flavor. During cancer treatment, as during regular life, it is important to be mindful of the bigger picture. Moderation is key.

During active treatment, your overall nutritional goal should be to eat a variety of foods that provide the nutrients needed to maintain health while fighting cancer. If you are having side effects that affect your ability to eat, talk with your oncologist. Advances have been made in the treatment of many side effects, and it is important you receive the appropriate treatment for your side effects. In addition to the treatment prescribed by your physician, there may be measures you can take to help with nutrition and eating problems. This book is about what you can do to help yourself during this time, not about what your doctor may prescribe. If you are having difficulty eating, you might ask your oncologist for a referral to see a registered dietitian who specializes in oncology nutrition. If one is not available at your clinic or medical center, contact the American Cancer Society at **800-227-2345** to request *Nutrition for the Person with Cancer During Treatment* or visit our Web site at **cancer.org** and click on "Patients,

Family, & Friends." You can also contact the American Dietetic Association (ADA) through their Web site (www.eatright.org). From www.eatright.org, click on "Find a Nutrition Professional" and put "Oncology Nutrition" in the expertise/specialty tab. You can also call the ADA at 800-877-1600 to identify a dietitian in your area.

How this Book Is Organized

This is not a typical cookbook. The recipes in this book are organized by side effect: nausea, diarrhea, constipation, sore mouth and difficulty swallowing, taste alterations, and unintentional weight loss. However, many of the recipes are applicable for people dealing with more than one side effect. As you're reading through the recipes, look for these symbols at the top of the page:

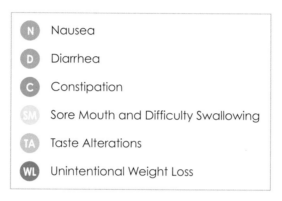

- **N** Nausea
- **D** Diarrhea
- **C** Constipation
- **SM** Sore Mouth and Difficulty Swallowing
- **TA** Taste Alterations
- **WL** Unintentional Weight Loss

This key also appears throughout the book. If an icon appears on the page with a given recipe, it means that the recipe would also be appropriate for that side effect. For example, the Minestrone Salad on page 47 appears in the chapter for constipation, but may also be appropriate if you are experiencing taste alterations, so both the **TA** and **C** icons appear on that page. We have also included that information in the list of recipes by symptom on pages viii–xii. Beside each recipe title, you'll see symbols that indicate whether that recipe is also appropriate for other side effects.

Most people with cancer have families who are sharing in the cancer experience. These recipes are intended not just for the person with cancer, but also for the family or caretaker to enjoy. While the recipes are focused on a cancer patient's specific needs, they are also nutritious and, for the most part, very easy and quick to prepare. Most incorporate ingredients you probably already have in your pantry. Since these recipes are written for people who are undergoing treatment, some are mildly flavored, and most make small portions. However, as you start to feel better or, depending on how you feel, you should feel free to adapt the recipes to suit your changing tastes. You may even want to use many of these recipes after you have finished your treatment.

How you eat while going through cancer treatment is different in many ways from how you might have eaten before. Many people going through cancer treatment experience a lack of appetite or other problems that can make eating daunting or difficult. A large plate of food can be overwhelming. It sometimes works better for those dealing with side effects to snack or eat small meals throughout the day. With those things in mind, we have deliberately made serving sizes fairly small. Keep in mind also that serving sizes are approximate—exact serving sizes will depend on the size of your ingredients (vegetables, for example) and your preparation.

Some of the recipes in the book have been adapted from other American Cancer Society publications. They have been tested and changed to best fit the needs of a person going through cancer treatment. Many of the recipes also include tips and suggestions to adapt them according to your needs—if you need to watch your weight, for example, or if you're trying to gain weight.

Three of us work as dietitians with the American Cancer Society, and we frequently speak with individuals who are going through treatment and dealing with side effects and nutritional challenges. Based on our experiences, we identified some of the most useful information to share in this book. On pages xvii-xviii, we offer advice for the caregiver. We recommend that caregivers read that section first. Taking care of someone who is going through cancer treatment can be very challenging, but also very rewarding. A Kitchen Staples list on pages 140–141 goes over some of the basics to keep on hand to be able to make many of the recipes included here. On page 142, we give a few tips to make dining out in a restaurant a bit easier. We also address the issue of excess weight gain (page 143), a problem that can affect many people going through cancer treatment.

Whether you need help dealing with side effects or simply want to make sure you maintain your health, this cookbook was written to help you. We hope that these recipes and our suggestions will make this time a little bit easier for everyone. Each person is different, and your cancer experience is unique. As mentioned earlier, there are no hard and fast rules about how to eat during cancer treatment. With trial and error, you can learn what works best for you.

For more information about cancer, nutrition, and managing the side effects of treatment, contact the American Cancer Society at 800-227-2345 or visit our Web site at cancer.org.

Advice for the Caregiver

Caregivers may find it frustrating and difficult to try to meet the nutritional needs of a family member or friend who may not want to eat at all or whose likes and dislikes may change on a daily basis.

When your loved one does not feel like eating, it is important to be patient and encouraging. Five or six small snacks a day may work better than three large meals. Don't worry if the person's diet is not as balanced as you would like; good days will make up for not-so-great days. Foods may not taste "normal" to someone going through cancer treatment, so don't be offended if old favorites aren't successful. If the person's tastes seem to have changed, encourage trying new foods. If an old favorite is not appealing, perhaps a new food will be surprisingly well received. Keep the fridge, freezer, and pantry stocked with easy-to-prepare convenience foods (see "Kitchen Staples" on pages 140–141). Put together a basket or cooler full of snacks your loved one can keep handy to nibble on when the urge strikes (see "The Survival Kit," page 139).

Here are some tips that you may find helpful:

- Prepare the biggest meal of the day when he or she feels the hungriest—often this may be in the morning.

- Offer favorite foods any time of the day. It's okay to have a sandwich or bowl of soup for breakfast or have breakfast food any time of day.

- Casseroles containing pasta, rice, and potatoes tend to be well tolerated. Many favorite casserole recipes can be easily altered to increase the amount of calories and protein they contain.

- Consider adding finely chopped meats, cheese, or hard-boiled eggs to soups, sauces, or casseroles for extra calories and protein.

- Spicy, greasy, or heavy foods may not be well tolerated on an unsettled stomach.

- Add sauces, broths, or cheese to foods to enhance flavor and ease swallowing if necessary.

- Package leftovers in single-serving containers for convenient re-serving later; large servings can seem overwhelming when the appetite is poor.

- If your loved one is sensitive to smells, prepare meals in a different room from where they'll be eaten. Consider grilling outdoors or using a slow cooker on the back porch or in the garage to keep the aroma of food from permeating the inside of the home. Suggest that the person go to another room or to the opposite side of the house while food is being prepared. Serving foods cool or at room temperature also helps to lessen smells.

- Your loved one may be hesitant to ask for help. Let the person know you want to assist in preparing meals or snacks, doing the food shopping, or handling other tasks.

- Drinking is often easier than eating. If the person does not feel like eating but is willing to drink, offer sips of hot cocoa, milk, milkshakes, smoothies, soups, and canned nutritional supplements. Soups can be sipped out of mugs and reheated as needed.

Cancer treatment may reduce the person's ability to fight off infections. If you are preparing meals for someone undergoing treatment, keep these tips in mind:

- Wash your hands before and after preparing meals.

- Meat, fish, poultry, and eggs should be thoroughly cooked.

- To avoid cross contamination, use different cutting boards for meats and vegetables and use a clean knife when cutting different foods.

- Check expiration dates on packaged food. If you are unsure about an item's freshness or its expiration date, don't use it.

- Wash all fruits and vegetables under cold running water before peeling or cutting, and avoid bruised or damaged produce.

- Keep hot foods hot and cold foods cold. Refrigerate leftovers within 2 hours of serving.

- Discard refrigerated leftovers after 3 days.

- Avoid foods from buffet lines and self-serve bulk bins.

- If your loved one is neutropenic or immunocompromised, ask the doctor for specific nutrition guidelines.

Chapter 1

NAUSEA

You may experience nausea and vomiting while you are going through cancer treatment. The occurrence of these side effects varies widely and depends on the person and the type of treatment received. Some people undergoing cancer treatment may have nausea and vomiting, whereas others may have only nausea. Many have neither.

The most common causes of nausea and vomiting are chemotherapy and radiation therapy to areas of the body such as the stomach, abdomen, and brain. If chemotherapy or radiation therapy is causing nausea or vomiting, controlling it with the proper medication is very important. If you are prescribed anti-nausea medication, take it as directed. Nausea is often easier to prevent than treat. If the medication does not relieve the nausea and/or vomiting, ask your physician whether a different medicine might be more beneficial. If you cannot keep the anti-nausea medication down, ask for one in suppository form. No matter the cause of your nausea or vomiting, this may be a time of trial and error as you and your doctor work to find the best way to deal with these side effects.

Dehydration can occur quite easily if you are vomiting. Though it may be difficult, try to sip small amounts of liquid every few minutes. You can suck on ice chips or juice bars to get fluids or sip liquids such as fruit juice, flat soda, slushies, water, cool broth, sports drinks, and tea. Once clear liquids stay down, you can add easy-to-digest foods such as crackers, toast, and dry cereals.

Your once-favorite foods may no longer be appealing, and food likes and dislikes can change frequently. Experiment with different foods and flavors to see what works for you.

The recipes in this chapter are designed to meet the needs of someone dealing with nausea. Many of the recipes make small, manageable portions or small, almost bite-sized foods. The flavors tend to be fairly mild. Many of the recipes are easy to serve at room temperature in order to minimize odors and tastes. We have also included recipes for drinks and slushies—things that will help keep you hydrated while also providing some nutrition. As nausea improves, it is easy to add more flavor to these recipes by including your favorite ingredients or increasing the amounts of spices used.

N	Nausea
D	Diarrhea
C	Constipation
SM	Sore Mouth and Difficulty Swallowing
TA	Taste Alterations
WL	Unintentional Weight Loss

Managing Nausea

- Eat a small, light meal or snack before chemotherapy and radiation treatments unless otherwise directed.

- Keep food in your stomach by eating small frequent snacks throughout the day. Snack ideas include smoothies, trail mix, fruit, or half of a sandwich.

- Try starchy foods such as pretzels, crackers, noodles, potatoes, bagels, dry cereals, bread-sticks, or rice.

- Try bland foods such as soups, smoothies, gelatin, and cream of wheat. Avoid fried, greasy, and rich foods.

- Suck on frozen fruit such as watermelon, peaches, grapes, strawberries, and cherries.

- Eat food cool or cold to decrease its smell and taste. Sometimes strong odors and flavors can trigger nausea.

- Do not take medications (especially pain medications) on an empty stomach unless the pharmacist directs otherwise.

- Don't eat your favorite foods when you don't feel well. If you consume your favorite foods during this difficult time, you may associate them with nausea and find them unappealing when treatment is over.

Managing Sensitivity to Smells

- Others may not be aware you are sensitive to smells or that they can trigger nausea. Don't hesitate to discuss which smells are offensive, for example, those of certain foods, perfume, cologne, air fresheners, or candles.

- Foods with strong odors may cause nausea and loss of appetite. If the smell of food being cooked is bothersome, ask others preparing food in your home to cook in a separate part of the house, grill outdoors, or use a slow cooker on the back porch or in the garage.

- Sipping broths and soups from insulated travel mugs with lids will help block odor (and help keep the liquid warm).

- To minimize the smell of canned nutritional supplements, try drinking them through a straw in a lidded cup.

- Try eating take-out or prepared foods instead of cooking for yourself. However, avoid eating at buffet-style restaurants or take-out foods from buffets.

- Cold, cool, or room-temperature foods will give off fewer odors than warm or hot foods. Chicken salad, fruit salads, yogurt, cold sandwiches, cereal, and deviled eggs are all good choices.

- Ask another person to cook for you. Ask that he or she remove any food covers to release food odors before entering your room or eating area.

For more information on managing nausea and vomiting,
call the American Cancer Society at 800-227-2345
or visit our Web site at cancer.org.

Lemon-Lime Smoothie

A balance of tart and sweet helps this smoothie go down easily. For a more tart flavor, choose plain yogurt instead of vanilla or add fresh lemon and/or lime juice. For stronger citrus flavor without the acidity, substitute lemon- or lime-flavored yogurt.

1 serving

Prep Time:
15 minutes or less

Total Time:
15 minutes or less

Nutritional Information
Per Serving
Calories 350
Total Fat . . . . 3.5 g
Total Carbohydrate . . . . . . 73 g
Dietary Fiber . . . . 0 g
Sugars . . . . 70 g
Protein . . . . 10 g
Sodium . . . . 160 mg

This recipe may not be appropriate if you have mouth sores.

5 to 6 ice cubes
1 cup vanilla or plain low-fat or nonfat yogurt
2 tablespoons frozen lemonade concentrate, partially thawed, but still icy
2 tablespoons frozen limeade concentrate, partially thawed, but still icy

1. In a blender, crush 5 ice cubes. Add the yogurt, lemonade, and limeade and blend until smooth. For a colder shake, add the remaining ice cube and blend until combined.

Chicken Noodle Soup

A store-bought rotisserie chicken is a mealtime lifesaver. It can be made into salads, sandwiches, or, as in this recipe, a classically loved soup.

This version uses all of the white breast meat from the chicken. Sautéing the wings and other bones with the aromatic vegetables adds richer flavor. If you prefer a less chunky soup, start with just 1 cup of chicken and add more to taste. If you want a thicker noodle-filled broth, increase the amount of noodles in the recipe by ½ cup. Unused dark meat can be saved for another meal.

8 servings

Prep Time:
15 minutes or less

Total Time:
1 hour or less

Nutritional Information
Per Serving (about 1 cup)
Calories 120
Total Fat . . . . 3.5 g
Total Carbohydrate . . . . 6 g
Dietary Fiber . . . . 1 g
Sugars . . . . 2 g
Protein . . . . 16 g
Sodium . . . . 420 mg

If your stomach is queasy, choose a rotisserie chicken with mild seasoning. Both traditional and lemon-pepper work well. If you are looking for stronger flavor, pick a spicier variety.

Avoid getting a rotisserie chicken that has been sitting out for a while. Try asking the deli staff whether they can give you a fresh one or tell you which are the freshest in the warmer.

1 rotisserie chicken full breast or 3 cups chopped cooked chicken
1 tablespoon vegetable oil
1 onion, chopped
1 large carrot (or 2 small), sliced
1 large celery stalk (or 2 small), sliced
6 cups reduced-sodium chicken broth
2 cups water
½ to 1 cup egg noodles
2 tablespoons chopped fresh Italian parsley
Salt and freshly ground black pepper

1. Remove the wings from the chicken breast and reserve. Remove the skin from the breast and discard. Shred the meat off the breastbone and break the breastbone into two pieces. Reserve the meat and bones separately.

2. In a stockpot over medium-high heat, add the oil. Sauté the onion, carrot, celery, chicken wings, and breastbone for 8 to 10 minutes, or until vegetables soften.

3. Add the broth and water and stir to combine. Bring to a boil. Reduce the heat, cover, and simmer for 15 to 20 minutes, stirring occasionally. Add the noodles and cook for 5 minutes, stirring occasionally. Add reserved chicken and parsley and cook for 2 to 3 minutes. Discard the bones before serving. Season with salt and pepper.

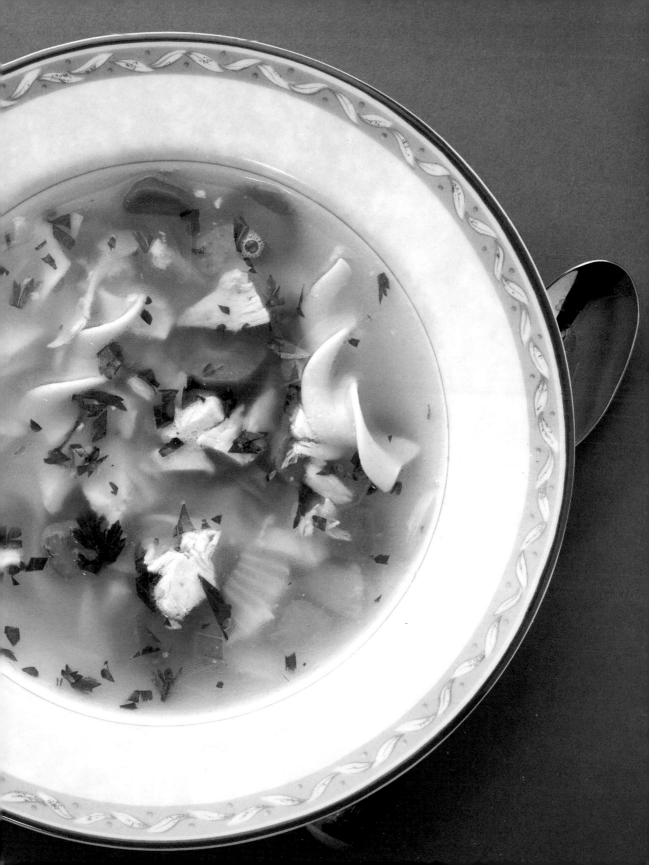

Ginger-Mint Tea

Ginger has long been thought to calm gastric distress. This recipe pairs ginger with mint tea for a soothing drink. Using an herbal mint tea allows you to enjoy this relaxing drink at any time, day or night.

1 serving

Prep Time:
15 minutes or less

Total Time:
15 minutes or less

**Nutritional Information
Per Serving**
Calories 70
Total Fat . . . . 0 g
Total Carbohydrate . . . . . . 18 g
Dietary Fiber . . . . 0 g
Sugars . . . . 17 g
Protein . . . . 0 g
Sodium . . . . 15 mg

For more acidic flavor, add 1 tablespoon of fresh lemon juice. For a sweeter drink, add more honey.

1 cup water
1 (1-inch) piece fresh ginger, peeled and thinly sliced
1 mint tea bag
1 tablespoon honey

1. In a saucepan over low heat, combine the water and ginger. Simmer for 5 minutes. Remove from heat, cover, and let steep for 5 minutes.

2. Strain into a mug and add the tea bag and honey. Let steep for another 3 to 5 minutes.

Mini Cheese Frittatas

Make these miniature frittatas—an egg dish that's similar to a baked omelet—in advance, and you can snack on them throughout the day. Reheat leftovers in the microwave for 12 to 15 seconds. If you're not in the mood for this filling, customize your own by using your favorite cheese, cooked meat, vegetable, or herb.

Eat as is, or sandwich a frittata inside a toasted English muffin for a heartier meal.

10 frittatas

Prep Time:
15 minutes or less

Total Time:
30 minutes or less

Nutritional Information
Per Serving (2 frittatas)
Calories 140
Total Fat . . . . 10 g
Total Carbohydrate . . . . 2 g
Dietary Fiber . . . . 0 g
Sugars . . . . 1 g
Protein . . . . 11 g
Sodium . . . . 160 mg

For added calories, choose whole milk or half-and-half and full-fat cheese. To reduce calories, use low-fat or reduced-fat options.

6 eggs
½ cup shredded regular or reduced-fat Cheddar or mozzarella cheese
¼ cup low-fat or whole milk or half-and-half
2 scallions, white and light green parts only, thinly sliced
Pinch dried thyme
Salt and freshly ground black pepper

1. Preheat the oven to 350 degrees. Generously coat a muffin tin with nonstick cooking spray.

2. In a bowl, beat the eggs. Add the cheese, milk, scallions, and thyme. Sprinkle with salt and pepper and stir well to combine. Spoon the mixture evenly into muffin cups.

3. Bake for 13 to 15 minutes, or until set. Leave in the tin for 1 minute before removing.

"On the Go" Snack Mix

Snack mixes are handy to have preassembled for a quick snack. Keep the mix in a tightly sealed container in the car or by the couch.

You can adapt the ingredients, depending on your symptoms. If you're experiencing constipation, include dried fruits and cereals with at least 5 grams of fiber, such as Mini Wheats, Crunchy Corn Bran, or Wheat Chex. A sprinkling of nuts adds protein. And, of course, a little chocolate rarely hurts!

9 servings

Prep Time:
15 minutes or less

Total Time:
15 minutes or less

Nutritional Information
Per Serving (about ½ cup)
Calories 145
Total Fat . . . . 7 g
Total Carbohydrate . . . . . . 19 g
Dietary Fiber . . . . 2 g
Sugars . . . . 7 g
Protein . . . . 4 g
Sodium . . . . 170 mg

Nuts provide protein
and are relatively low
in saturated fat.

1 cup pretzels
1 cup peanut butter Ritz bits, Wheat Thins, or other small crackers
**1 cup whole grain cereal, such as Cheerios or Quaker Oatmeal
   Squares**
½ cup almonds (dry roasted)
½ cup raisins
½ cup plain or peanut M&Ms, optional

1. In a container with an airtight lid, combine the pretzels, crackers, cereal, almonds, raisins, and M&Ms.

Twice-Baked Potatoes

Twice-baked potatoes transform a standard baked potato into a creamy and comforting small meal. The potato skin becomes an edible shell for mildly flavored mashed potatoes, the ultimate comfort food.

For a more substantial meal, keep the potatoes whole instead of halving them. Slice a ½ inch off the top of each potato lengthwise and hollow out the skins. For stronger flavor, top with minced fresh chives or additional Parmesan cheese.

If you're trying to increase calories, add butter, substitute heavy cream for the milk, and choose full-fat cheeses. If you're trying to control your weight, choose reduced-fat options.

Instead of being microwaved, the potatoes can also be baked for 1 hour at 350 degrees.

4 servings

Prep Time:
15 minutes or less

Total Time:
45 minutes or less

Nutritional Information
Per Serving
Calories 205
Total Fat . . . . 6 g
Total Carbohydrate . . . . . . 33 g
Dietary Fiber . . . . 3 g
Sugars . . . . 1 g
Protein . . . . 5 g
Sodium . . . . 70 mg

2 large (12 to 14 ounces) Russet potatoes, scrubbed
1 tablespoon butter, room temperature
2 to 3 tablespoons low-fat milk
2 to 3 tablespoons regular or reduced-fat sour cream
2 to 3 tablespoons regular or reduced-fat shredded Cheddar cheese
Salt and freshly ground black pepper
1 tablespoon grated Parmesan cheese

1. Pierce potatoes in several places with a fork. Microwave on high for 6 to 8 minutes, turning halfway through the cooking time if your microwave does not have a carousel or tends to heat unevenly. Remove and set aside to cool briefly.

2. Preheat the oven to 375 degrees.

3. When potatoes are cool enough to handle (but still very warm), cut them in half lengthwise and scoop the potato flesh into a mixing bowl, leaving a ¼-inch-thick shell and using care not to break the skins.

4. In the bowl with the potato flesh, add the butter and mash to combine. Add 2 tablespoons each of the milk, sour cream, and Cheddar cheese and mash until creamy and combined. Season with salt and pepper. Taste and add more milk, sour cream, or Cheddar cheese if necessary. Divide the mixture evenly among the potato shells. Arrange stuffed potatoes on a baking sheet and sprinkle with Parmesan cheese.

5. Bake for 15 to 20 minutes, or until cheese has melted and potatoes are lightly golden.

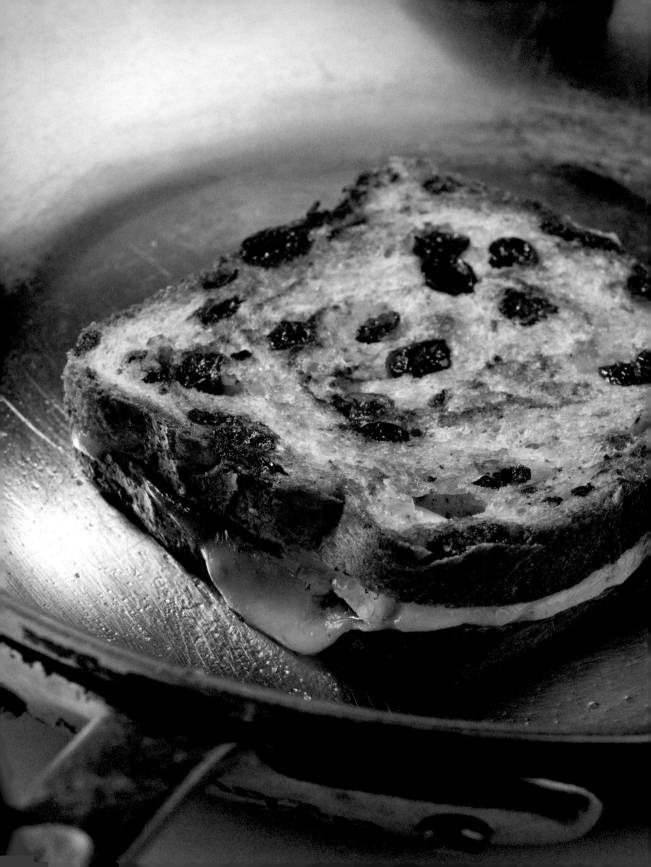

Brie and Apple Grilled Cheese

Sometimes a slight twist, like a special bread or an unexpected cheese, makes an ordinary sandwich suddenly appealing. In this heated sandwich, Brie, a creamy, soft cheese, melts into a yummy puddle of comfort on raisin bread.

You can substitute Cheddar or another hard cheese for Brie if your doctor has advised you to avoid soft cheeses.

1 serving

Prep Time:
15 minutes or less

Total Time:
15 minutes or less

**Nutritional Information
Per Serving**
Calories 310
Total Fat . . . . 17 g
Total Carbohydrate . . . . . . 30 g
Dietary Fiber . . . . 2 g
Sugars . . . . 9 g
Protein . . . . 10 g
Sodium . . . . 540 mg

Don't like raisins? You can substitute cinnamon swirl or any soft bread for the raisin bread in this sandwich.

**1½ ounces Brie cheese, white rind trimmed, or other cheese,
    at room temperature**
2 slices raisin bread
2 to 3 thin slices peeled Granny Smith or other apple
1 teaspoon butter, softened

1. Spread the Brie on one side of each piece of bread. Place apple on top of one slice and top with the other slice, cheese side down. Spread the butter on the other sides of the bread.

2. Place in a skillet over medium heat. Cook until the bottom is golden and the cheese begins to melt. Carefully turn the sandwich and cook until golden and the cheese has melted completely.

Cheese and Spinach Strata

Strata, a savory breakfast bread pudding, can be prepared the night before so the egg mixture has time to absorb into the bread, making a soft, custardy, comforting dish. Even though some people may be turned off by eggs, in this mild strata the egg flavor is not assertive.

This version includes chopped spinach for added nutrients, but you can leave it out if spinach isn't appealing. You can make the flavors stronger by adding sautéed mushrooms, tomatoes, or other ingredients if your stomach is up to it.

Use any type of leftover bread. For better texture, leave the bread out for several hours to go stale so the eggs will better soak into the bread.

6 to 8 servings

Prep Time:
30 minutes or less

Total Time:
1 hour and 30 minutes
plus 8 hours or more
refrigeration

Nutritional Information
Per Serving

Calories	250
Total Fat	12 g
Total Carbohydrate	20 g
Dietary Fiber	2 g
Sugars	5 g
Protein	16 g
Sodium	400 mg

Spinach is full of vitamins C, E, and K, as well as beta carotene, folate, and riboflavin. Eggs are not only high in protein, but also provide biotin, a structural component in bone and hair.

Reserve 1/4 cup of the spinach to make the Cheese and Spinach Portobello Pizzas (page 127).

5 eggs
1½ cups low-fat milk
5 cups cubed stale bread (about 1-inch cubes)
1 cup regular or reduced-fat shredded Cheddar cheese
1 (10-ounce) box frozen chopped spinach, thawed, squeezed of excess liquid, and patted dry
Salt and freshly ground black pepper

1. Generously coat an 8-by-8-inch baking pan with nonstick cooking spray.

2. In a large bowl, beat the eggs. Add the milk and stir well to combine. Add the bread, cheese, spinach, and season with salt and pepper and stir well to combine. Transfer to the baking dish. Cover with plastic wrap, pressing down to submerge the bread, and refrigerate overnight or for at least 2 hours.

3. When ready to bake, preheat the oven to 350 degrees. Remove the plastic wrap and cover tightly with foil.

4. Bake for 40 minutes. Remove the foil and bake for an additional 10 to 15 minutes, or until a knife inserted in the center comes out clean and the strata looks puffy. Let cool for 5 to 10 minutes before serving.

Baked Apples with Sugar and Cinnamon

This simple dessert has a mild taste and is easy to prepare. For more flavor, you can add ¹/₄ cup raisins or chopped nuts to the filling or sprinkle the apples with crumbled ginger snap cookies. If tolerated, consider adding ¹/₈ teaspoon of grated lemon zest to the filling to add an extra dimension of flavor.

The apples can be served warm or cold. If you have leftovers, make homemade applesauce by puréeing the apples and their cooking liquid in a food processor. Applesauce makes a great snack or can be enjoyed as a topping on angel food cake or with yogurt for breakfast.

4 servings

Prep Time:
15 minutes or less

Total Time:
1 hour and 30 minutes or less

**Nutritional Information
Per Serving (1 apple)**
Calories 160
Total Fat . . . . 0 g
Total Carbohydrate . . . . . . 42 g
Dietary Fiber . . . . 5 g
Sugars . . . . 35 g
Protein . . . . 1 g
Sodium . . . . 10 mg

To easily core apples and cut away the flesh around the core, use a curved grapefruit knife, serrated grapefruit spoon, or melon baller.

4 large Granny Smith or Golden Delicious apples
¹/₄ cup (packed) light brown sugar
¹/₂ teaspoon ground cinnamon
³/₄ cup boiling water

1. Preheat the oven to 375 degrees.

2. Peel the skin from the top quarter of the apples. Core apples, leaving ¹/₂ inch of core at the bottom, using care not to puncture the bottoms and sides.

3. In a bowl, combine the brown sugar and cinnamon and fill the apples with the mixture. Place apples cavity side up in an 8-by-8-inch baking pan and pour boiling water around the apples.

4. Bake for 60 minutes, occasionally basting the apples with juices from the pan. Let cool for 5 to 10 minutes before serving, basting occasionally.

Adapted, with permission, from *Eating Well, Staying Well During and After Cancer* (Atlanta, GA: American Cancer Society, 2004), 235.

Pineapple-Mango Slushies

To make this easy, frosty treat, simply freeze a juice and fruit mixture and, right before serving, purée in the food processor until it has a soft and slushy texture.

You can also use this recipe to make fruit pops. Cover each paper cup with a piece of plastic wrap or aluminum foil and make a slit in the wrap. Insert a plastic spoon or Popsicle stick through the wrap and freeze until the fruit mixture is solid, at least 3 hours.

4 servings

Prep Time:
15 minutes or less

Total Time:
**15 minutes or less plus
3 or more hours freezing**

**Nutritional Information
Per Serving (about 1 cup)**
Calories 125
Total Fat . . . . 0 g
Total Carbohydrate . . . . . . 30 g
Dietary Fiber . . . . 1 g
Sugars . . . . 30 g
Protein . . . . 0 g
Sodium . . . . 25 mg

You can use any flavor of juice that sounds appealing or try other fruits in place of the pineapple, such as kiwi or berries.

This recipe is not appropriate if you have mouth sores.

1 (8-ounce) can crushed pineapple in juice

3 cups mango-pineapple or other tropical fruit juice, divided

1. In four ($^3/_4$- to 1-cup) paper cups, divide pineapple evenly (about $^1/_4$ cup per cup). Fill each cup with $^1/_2$ cup juice and stir to combine. Cover each cup with plastic wrap and freeze until solid, at least 3 hours.

2. Remove the frozen mixture from the cups by running the outside of each cup under hot water and peeling off the paper. Place the frozen pops (one at a time) in a food processor with $^1/_4$ cup juice and process until slushy.

Homemade Berry Frozen Yogurt

Creamy, refreshing frozen yogurt is just a few moments away when using a food processor. Keep bags of fruit in the freezer for times when a sweet, cool treat sounds like the perfect thing.

6 servings

Prep Time:
15 minutes or less

Total Time:
15 minutes or less

Nutritional Information
Per Serving
Calories 75
Total Fat . . . . 0 g
Total Carbohydrate . . . . . . 18 g
Dietary Fiber . . . . 2 g
Sugars . . . . 14 g
Protein . . . . 2 g
Sodium . . . . 20 mg

1 (16-ounce) package frozen strawberries or other berries
1 (6-ounce) container plain nonfat or low-fat yogurt
⅓ cup plus 2 tablespoons confectioners sugar

1. Defrost the strawberries in a microwave oven on 30 percent power for 45 seconds to 1 minute. They should still feel frozen.

2. In a food processor, combine the berries, yogurt, and confectioners sugar and process until smooth. Serve immediately.

Adapted, with permission, from *The Great American Eat-Right Cookbook* (Atlanta, GA: American Cancer Society, 2007), 183.

Pumpkin-Ginger Mini Muffins

These delicately spiced muffins get extra flavor and texture from currants (perfectly sized for miniature treats) and crystallized ginger, available in the baking section of most supermarkets. To make these muffins extra mild, you can leave out the crystallized ginger.

24 mini muffins

Prep Time:
15 minutes or less

Total Time:
30 minutes or less

**Nutritional Information
Per Serving (1 mini muffin)**
Calories 65
Total Fat . . . . 2 g
Total Carbohydrate . . . . . . 11 g
Dietary Fiber . . . . 0 g
Sugars . . . . 6 g
Protein . . . . 1 g
Sodium . . . . 70 mg

For stronger flavor, increase the amounts of the ground spices.

Use leftover pumpkin in Pumpkin Custard (page 68) or the Pumpkin Shake (page 70).

To make regular-sized muffins, add 5 to 10 minutes to the baking time. This recipe makes about a dozen regular-sized muffins.

1 cup all-purpose flour
1/2 cup granulated sugar
1 teaspoon baking powder
1/4 teaspoon baking soda
1/4 teaspoon salt
1/2 teaspoon ground cinnamon
1/2 teaspoon ground ginger
Pinch ground nutmeg
Pinch ground cloves
1/4 cup currants, golden raisins, or brown raisins
2 tablespoons finely chopped crystallized ginger
1 egg
1/4 cup butter, melted and slightly cooled
3 tablespoons water
1/2 cup canned pumpkin purée

1. Preheat the oven to 350 degrees. Coat two mini muffin tins with nonstick cooking spray or fill with paper liners.

2. In a bowl, combine flour, sugar, baking powder, baking soda, salt, cinnamon, ground ginger, nutmeg, and cloves. Add the currants and crystallized ginger and stir gently to coat.

3. In a separate bowl, beat the egg. Add the butter, water, and pumpkin and stir to combine. Add the egg mixture to the dry ingredients and gently stir to incorporate. Spoon the batter evenly into muffin cups.

4. Bake for 12 to 15 minutes, or until the tops just bounce back when touched. Leave in the tins for 5 minutes before transferring to a cooling rack.

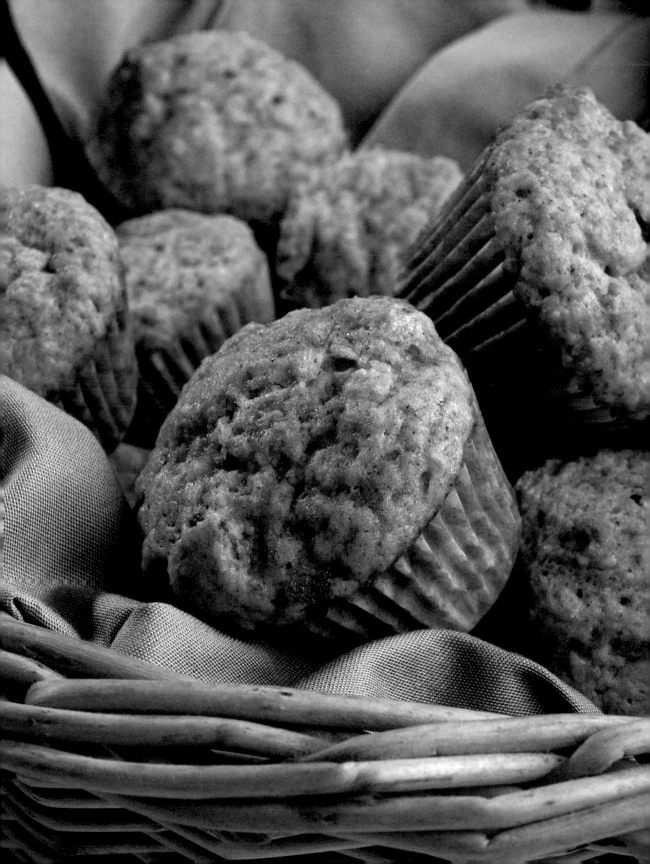

Cinnamon-Sugar French Toast Fingers

These soft and puffy miniature slices of French toast can be prepared ahead of time and reheated before eating. To make this French toast more finger food–friendly, the bread is cut into strips and sweetened with a sprinkle of cinnamon-sugar (instead of syrup) after cooking.

Choose soft, flavorful bread like a raisin loaf or a challah that you can slice a little thicker than standard sandwich bread. Thick slices can soak up the egg mixture and still keep their shape.

2 servings

Prep Time:
15 minutes or less

Total Time:
30 minutes or less

**Nutritional Information
Per Serving (3 "fingers")**
Calories 245
Total Fat . . . . 11 g
Total Carbohydrate . . . . . . 28 g
Dietary Fiber . . . . 1 g
Sugars . . . . 17 g
Protein . . . . 9 g
Sodium . . . . 340 mg

Make your own cinnamon-sugar by combining 1/4 cup granulated sugar with 1 tablespoon ground cinnamon. Store in an airtight container.

For added calories, substitute half-and-half or whole milk for the low-fat milk.

2 eggs
1/2 cup low-fat milk
2 tablespoons granulated sugar
1/2 teaspoon vanilla extract
1/2 teaspoon ground cinnamon
1/4 teaspoon ground nutmeg
1/8 teaspoon salt
2 slices raisin or other bread, cut into thirds
1 tablespoon butter
1/4 teaspoon cinnamon-sugar

1. In a bowl, beat the eggs. Add the milk, sugar, vanilla, cinnamon, nutmeg, and salt and stir well to combine. Add the bread and coat with egg mixture, turning the pieces if necessary. Let the bread soak for 5 minutes or until much of the mixture has been absorbed.

2. In a large skillet or griddle over medium heat, melt the butter. Add the bread, letting excess liquid drip off, and cook for 3 to 4 minutes per side, or until golden. Remove to a plate and sprinkle with cinnamon-sugar.

Creamy Rice Pudding

This classic dish is the chicken soup of desserts. It can usually make you feel better, regardless of the symptom. This version tastes rich and lush but is actually made with low-fat milk and no eggs or cream. As the mixture cooks, the rice gradually absorbs the milk, becoming thick and creamy.

The pudding needs to be stirred frequently, but otherwise requires little effort. It can easily be prepared while you are in the kitchen getting dinner or lunch ready.

After most of the milk has evaporated, monitor the rice closely, stirring constantly and tasting for tenderness. Add milk as necessary until the pudding is velvety and the rice is soft but still has some texture.

If desired, add raisins, dried cherries, or other dried fruit. For added flavor, increase the amount of finely grated lemon or orange zest to 1 teaspoon.

This version is not cloyingly sweet. However, if you are sensitive to sweets, reduce the sugar to ¹/₄ cup and add more to taste midway through cooking if necessary.

4 servings

Prep Time:
15 minutes or less

Total Time:
1 hour or less

**Nutritional Information
Per Serving**
Calories 230
Total Fat . . . . 2 g
Total Carbohydrate . . . . . . 44 g
Dietary Fiber . . . . 0 g
Sugars . . . . 26 g
Protein . . . . 8 g
Sodium . . . . 115 mg

If your mouth is very sensitive, add milk until the rice is very soft and omit the dried fruit and lemon or orange zest.

For added flavor, increase the amount of zest used.

¹/₂ **cup white rice or Arborio rice**

3 to 4 cups low-fat milk

¹/₃ **cup granulated sugar**

¹/₂ **teaspoon finely grated lemon or orange zest, optional**

Pinch salt

1 teaspoon vanilla extract

¹/₃ **cup raisins or dried cherries, optional**

Ground cinnamon

1. In a large saucepan over medium heat, bring the rice, 3 cups of the milk, sugar, zest, and salt to a simmer, stirring occasionally. Reduce the heat and keep the mixture at a gentle simmer for 35 to 40 minutes, stirring frequently, until the pudding thickens and the rice is tender. If the milk begins to form a skin on the surface of the pudding, just stir it in. If the pudding thickens and the rice is still too firm, add more milk ¹/₄ cup at a time, until absorbed and the rice softens.

2. Add the vanilla and raisins and cook for an additional 5 to 10 minutes, or until creamy and tender, stirring constantly. Serve warm or transfer to individual bowls and chill. Just before serving, sprinkle with cinnamon.

Zucchini Bites

These baked treats are a great little snack, appetizer, or side dish. The zucchini stays soft and melts in your mouth, while the coating provides a little crunch without the greasiness of frying.

If the Parmesan cheese makes you feel nauseated, substitute a less pungent cheese or omit the cheese altogether.

4 to 6 servings

Prep Time:
15 minutes or less

Total Time:
30 minutes or less

Nutritional Information
Per serving
Calories 75
Total Fat . . . . 2.5 g
Total Carbohydrate . . . . . . 10 g
Dietary Fiber . . . . 1 g
Sugars . . . . 3 g
Protein . . . . 5 g
Sodium . . . . 350 mg

$\frac{1}{4}$ **cup regular or whole wheat pancake mix**
2 tablespoons grated Parmesan cheese
$\frac{1}{2}$ **teaspoon garlic salt**
$\frac{1}{2}$ **teaspoon paprika**
1 egg
2 medium zucchini, cut into $\frac{3}{4}$-inch slices

1. Preheat the oven to 350 degrees. Line a rimmed baking sheet with foil and lightly coat with nonstick cooking spray.

2. On a plate, combine the pancake mix, Parmesan cheese, garlic salt, and paprika. In a bowl, beat the egg. Dip the zucchini in egg, then coat with the pancake mix, shaking off the excess, and place on the baking sheet.

3. Bake for 7 to 10 minutes and then turn over. Bake for an additional 7 to 8 minutes, or until golden.

Adapted, with permission, from *Celebrate! Healthy Entertaining for Any Occasion* (Atlanta, GA: American Cancer Society, 2001), 40.

Blueberry-Corn Mini Muffins

These not-too-sweet muffins get antioxidants through the addition of blueberries. If using frozen berries, use small ones and do not defrost first.

Coating the blueberries with flour keeps them more evenly dispersed in the batter.

24 mini muffins

Prep Time:
15 minutes or less

Total Time:
30 minutes or less

Nutritional Information
Per Serving (1 mini muffin)
Calories 55
Total Fat . . . . 2.5 g
Total Carbohydrate . . . . 7 g
Dietary Fiber . . . . 0 g
Sugars . . . . 3 g
Protein . . . . 1 g
Sodium . . . . 80 mg

If you don't have canola oil on hand, you can substitute another vegetable oil.

To make regular-sized muffins, add 5 to 10 minutes to the baking time. This recipe should make about twelve regular-sized muffins.

$^3/_4$ **cup cornmeal**
$^1/_4$ **cup all-purpose flour**
3 tablespoons granulated sugar
1$^1/_4$ teaspoons baking powder
$^1/_2$ **teaspoon salt**
1 cup fresh or frozen blueberries
1 egg
$^3/_4$ **cup buttermilk**
$^1/_4$ **cup canola oil**

1. Preheat the oven to 400 degrees. Coat two mini muffin tins with nonstick cooking spray or fill with paper liners.

2. In a bowl, combine the cornmeal, flour, sugar, baking powder, and salt. Add the blueberries and stir gently to coat.

3. In a separate bowl, beat the egg. Add the buttermilk and oil and stir to combine. Add the egg mixture to the dry ingredients and stir gently to incorporate. Spoon the batter evenly into muffin cups.

4. Bake for 15 to 17 minutes, or until the tops just bounce back when touched. Leave in the tins for 5 minutes before transferring to a cooling rack.

Beef and Vegetable-Barley Soup

This hearty, chunky soup is a great way to satisfy a red meat craving while getting healthy vegetables and grains at the same time.

11 servings

Prep Time:
30 minutes or less

Total Time:
1 hour and 15 minutes
or less

Per Serving (about 1 cup)
Calories 110
Total Fat . . . . 3 g
Total Carbohydrate . . . . . . 11 g
Dietary Fiber . . . . 2 g
Sugars . . . . 2 g
Protein . . . . 10 g
Sodium . . . . 380 mg

1 tablespoon olive oil
1 pound lean stew beef, cut into ½-inch pieces
1 small (or ½ large) onion, chopped
1 celery stalk, chopped
1 carrot, chopped
1 garlic clove, finely chopped
7 cups reduced-sodium beef broth
1 (14.5-ounce) can diced tomatoes
½ teaspoon dried basil
1 bay leaf
½ cup barley
Salt and freshly ground black pepper

1. In a stockpot over medium-high heat, add the oil. Brown the beef on all sides. Remove the beef and set aside. You may need to brown the beef in two or more batches, depending on the size of your skillet.

2. Add the onion, celery, and carrot to the stockpot and sauté for 5 to 8 minutes, or until softened. Add the garlic and sauté for 1 minute. Add the broth, tomatoes, basil, and bay leaf and stir to combine. Bring to a boil. Add the barley and reserved beef and stir to combine. Reduce the heat, partially cover, and simmer for 50 minutes, stirring occasionally. Season with salt and pepper. Remove the bay leaf before serving.

Adapted, with permission, from *Eating Well, Staying Well During and After Cancer* (Atlanta, GA: American Cancer Society, 2004), 220.

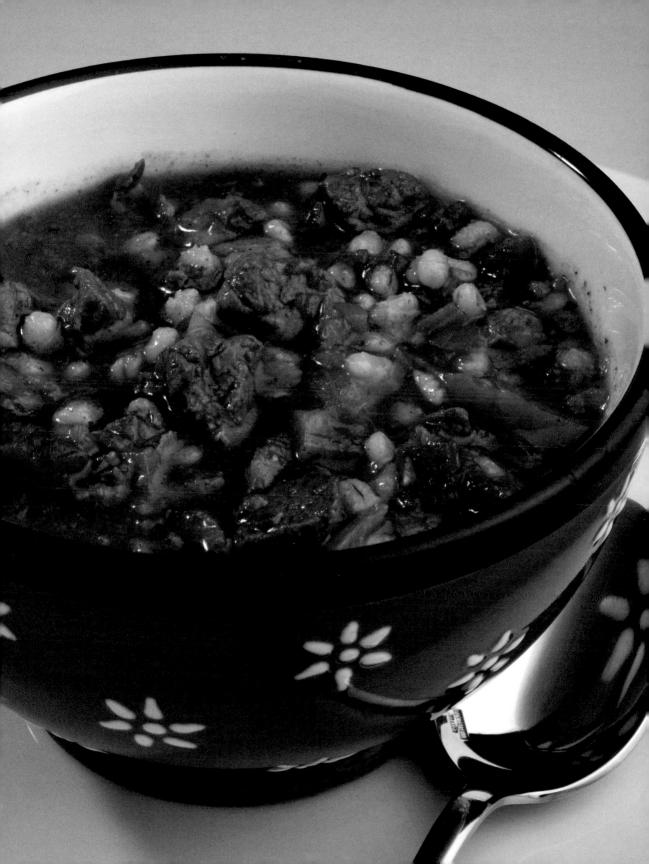

Spiced Hot Cider

When you are looking for liquid calories but don't want a shake, try this spiced cider. Refrigerate extra spiced cider and reheat when needed.

4 servings

Prep Time:
15 minutes or less

Total Time:
15 minutes or less

Nutritional Information
Per Serving (about 1 cup)
Calories 130
Total Fat . . . . 0 g
Total Carbohydrate . . . . . . 33 g
Dietary Fiber . . . . 1 g
Sugars . . . . 29 g
Protein . . . . 0 g
Sodium . . . . 10 mg

4 cups pasteurized apple cider
6 cloves
5 allspice berries
1 cinnamon stick
1 (1-inch) piece fresh ginger, thinly sliced
1 orange, sliced
1 to 2 tablespoons honey

1. In a saucepan over low heat, combine the cider, cloves, allspice, cinnamon stick, ginger, orange slices, and 1 table-spoon of the honey. Simmer for 8 to 10 minutes.

2. Strain into mugs. Taste and add the remaining tablespoon of honey if necessary.

Very hot beverages can sometimes be irritating to the stomach. If that is the case for you, let this drink cool to room temperature before drinking.

This cider is a good choice for patients advised not to drink cold beverages because of the type of chemotherapy they are receiving.

Chapter 2

Diarrhea can be caused by a number of factors. Chemotherapy drugs may damage the rapidly dividing cells of the digestive tract. Radiation to the prostate, cervix, intestine, rectum, or pancreas and surgery to the stomach, intestine, or pancreas may alter digestion and absorption. If left untreated, ongoing diarrhea can lead to dehydration, weight loss, poor appetite, decreased strength and energy, and electrolyte imbalances. Talk to your doctor if you experience diarrhea so that appropriate treatment can be prescribed. Treatment will be based on the cause of the diarrhea. For example, your doctor may recommend a different treatment for diarrhea that is caused by radiation therapy to the abdomen than for diarrhea caused by chemotherapy.

Be sure to sip clear fluids throughout the day to prevent dehydration. One exception is apple juice, which may worsen diarrhea. When your diarrhea starts to improve, begin eating small amounts of low-fiber, easy-to-digest foods, such as white rice, bananas, applesauce, low-fat yogurt, mashed potatoes, and dry toast. If you are able to consume only clear liquids for 3 consecutive days, consult your oncology team for further recommendations.

In addition to any treatment your physician may prescribe for the diarrhea, there are several other things you can try to lessen diarrhea.

Managing Diarrhea

- Remain hydrated by drinking a cup of liquid after each loose stool. Sports drinks, bouillon or broth, diluted juices, fruit ice, Popsicles, or gelatin can help replace electrolytes and provide fluids. Room-temperature beverages may be easier to tolerate than cold or hot liquids. The majority of the beverages you drink should be caffeine free.

- Applesauce, bananas, canned peaches or pears, oatmeal, and white rice or pasta are easy to digest and may help to thicken stool.

(N)	Nausea
(D)	Diarrhea
(C)	Constipation
(SM)	Sore Mouth and Difficulty Swallowing
(TA)	Taste Alterations
(WL)	Unintentional Weight Loss

Soluble fiber helps to bind water in the stool. It can be found in oats, peeled apples, bananas, and psyllium husk. Soluble fiber has the added benefit of helping reduce cholesterol.

- Replace sodium in your diet through foods and drinks such as pretzels, crackers, soups, broths, and sports drinks.

- Replace potassium in your diet with bananas, potatoes (without the skins to decrease fiber), and sports drinks.

- Small, frequent meals may be easier to digest than larger meals.

- Limit dairy products to no more than 2 cups a day, as lactose can aggravate diarrhea. Dairy products with live and active cultures (such as buttermilk, yogurt, and kefir—a fermented milk drink) may be easier to digest. Avoid yogurt that is marketed to promote regularity.

- Avoid high-fiber foods like beans, peas, whole grains, and raw fruits and vegetables with the peel or skin left on.

- Avoid greasy, fried, spicy, or very sweet foods, which can irritate the digestive tract.

- Avoid sugar-free foods containing sugar alcohols such as maltitol, mannitol, sorbitol, lactitol, and xylitol, which can aggravate diarrhea.

- If diarrhea persists, contact your health care provider.

For more information about managing diarrhea, call the American Cancer Society at 800-227-2345 or visit our Web site at cancer.org.

Brown Sugar–Oatmeal Muffins

Heart-healthy oats give these mildly flavored muffins extra nutrients and provide binding action for those suffering from diarrhea. Soaking the oats in buttermilk helps soften them. For added flavor, increase the amount of cinnamon used.

12 muffins

Prep Time:
30 minutes or less

Total Time:
1 hour or less

**Nutritional Information
Per Serving (1 muffin)**
Calories 180
Total Fat . . . . 8 g
Total Carbohydrate . . . . . . 25 g
Dietary Fiber . . . . 1 g
Sugars . . . . 12 g
Protein . . . . 4 g
Sodium . . . . 220 mg

These muffins freeze well. Use just what you need and freeze the other muffins, defrosting one when you want something a little sweet.

With a few additions, these muffins are also a good option if you are experiencing constipation. Just add dried fruit, a chopped apple or pear, or nuts for additional fiber.

1 cup old-fashioned rolled oats
1 cup low-fat buttermilk
1 cup all-purpose flour
1 teaspoon baking powder
³/₄ teaspoon ground cinnamon
½ teaspoon baking soda
½ teaspoon salt
2 eggs
½ cup (packed) light brown sugar
½ cup applesauce
⅓ cup canola oil
1 teaspoon vanilla extract

1. Preheat the oven to 400 degrees. Coat a muffin tin with nonstick cooking spray or fill with paper liners.

2. In a bowl, combine the oats and buttermilk. Set aside for 25 minutes.

3. Meanwhile, in a bowl, combine the flour, baking powder, cinnamon, baking soda, and salt.

4. In a separate bowl, beat the eggs. Add the brown sugar, applesauce, oil, and vanilla and stir to combine. Add to the oat mixture, stirring well to combine. Add the dry ingredients and stir gently to incorporate. Spoon the batter evenly into muffin cups.

5. Bake for 13 to 18 minutes, or until the tops just bounce back when touched. Leave in the tin for 5 minutes before transferring to a cooling rack.

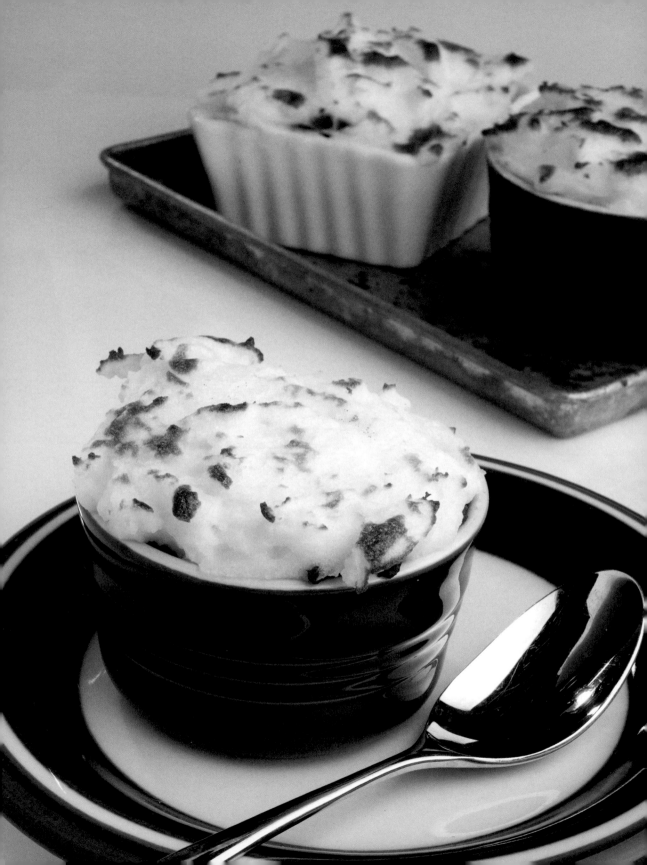

Mini Shepherd's Pies

These little pies are a meal unto themselves, providing meat, potatoes, and vegetables all in one bite. Mildly seasoned ground beef is topped with a mashed potato "crust" and baked in individual portions. Keep extras in the fridge to heat up during the week. To save time, you can use leftover mashed potatoes (about 2 cups' worth) or buy premade mashed potatoes. While this recipe contains peas, the small amount should not aggravate diarrhea.

You will need four ramekins or oven-safe teacups for this recipe.

4 servings

Prep Time:
15 minutes or less

Total Time:
45 minutes or less

Nutritional Information
Per Serving (1 pie)
Calories 380
Total Fat . . . . 17 g
Total Carbohydrate . . . . . . 30 g
Dietary Fiber . . . . 3 g
Sugars . . . . 7 g
Protein . . . . 26 g
Sodium . . . . 390 mg

Shepherd's pie can be baked in a larger dish for family-style eating. An 8-by-8-inch pan or round casserole dish should suffice. Bake for an additional 10 to 15 minutes, until the potatoes are golden.

Extra potatoes can be used in Mashed Potato–Chicken Patties (page 34).

If you're no longer having diarrhea, there's no need to peel the potatoes and lose their nutrients—just scrub well.

1 pound potatoes, peeled and cut into 2-inch pieces
2 tablespoons butter
2 to 4 tablespoons low-fat milk
Salt
1 tablespoon vegetable oil
1 pound lean ground beef
1 small (or ½ large) onion, finely chopped
⅓ cup ketchup
1 teaspoon Worcestershire sauce
1 cup frozen peas and carrots mixture

1. Preheat the oven to 400 degrees.

2. Fill a large saucepan with enough water to cover the potatoes by an inch or more and bring to a boil. Reduce to a simmer and cook until potatoes are tender. Drain and return to the pan. Add the butter and 2 tablespoons of the milk and mash until soft and creamy, adding more milk if necessary. Season with salt.

3. Meanwhile, in a large skillet over medium high heat, add the oil. Sauté the ground beef and onion for 6 to 8 minutes, or until meat is cooked through, stirring frequently to break up the meat. Drain if needed. Add the ketchup and Worcestershire sauce and stir well to combine. Add the peas and carrots and stir well to combine.

4. Divide meat mixture evenly between four (1-cup) ramekins or oven-safe teacups. Top with about ½ cup mashed potato, spreading to cover the meat. Place the ramekins on a baking sheet.

5. Bake for 10 minutes, or until the tops are golden. Let cool for 5 to 10 minutes before serving.

Baked Rice Balls

These mild baked nuggets of rice are simple enough to appeal even when you're feeling fragile. Adding Italian seasoning and using a stronger flavored cheese, such as Parmesan, perks them up a little. For added flavor, family members can dip them in pasta sauce.

Make extra rice the night before to use for these balls.

15 balls

Prep Time:
30 minutes or less

Total Time:
45 minutes or less

Nutritional Information
Per Serving (about 3 rice balls)
Calories 115
Total Fat . . . . 3 g
Total Carbohydrate . . . . . . 16 g
Dietary Fiber . . . . 0 g
Sugars . . . . 0 g
Protein . . . . 6 g
Sodium . . . . 85 mg

1 egg
1½ cups cooked white rice
½ cup grated or shredded mozzarella, Parmesan, or other cheese
2 tablespoons all-purpose flour
Salt and freshly ground black pepper
Pinch dried Italian seasoning, optional
1 cup pasta sauce, heated, optional

1. Preheat the oven to 350 degrees. Line a rimmed baking sheet with foil and lightly coat with nonstick cooking spray.

2. In a bowl, beat the egg. Add the rice, cheese, and flour and stir to combine. Sprinkle with salt, pepper, and Italian seasoning.

3. With wet hands, form the mixture into 1½-inch balls and place on the baking sheet. You may need to rewet your hands after every two to three balls.

4. Bake for 20 to 25 minutes, or until lightly golden. Serve with pasta sauce.

Fruity Gelatin

For delicate stomachs and sensitive mouths, a gelatin mold fits the bill, providing hydration and calories. Don't use apple juice or a tropical fruit mix—both could aggravate diarrhea.

8 servings

Prep Time:
15 minutes or less

Total Time:
15 minutes or less plus
5 or more hours
refrigeration

**Nutritional Information
Per Serving**
Calories 125
Total Fat . . . . 0 g
Total Carbohydrate . . . . . . 30 g
Dietary Fiber . . . . 1 g
Sugars . . . . 28 g
Protein . . . . 1 g
Sodium . . . . 85 mg

Choose your favorite
flavor of gelatin and
your favorite canned
fruit and fruit juice.

2 (3-ounce, 4-serving) boxes flavored gelatin
2 cups boiling water
1 (15-ounce) can mixed fruit in 100 percent juice
3/4 to 1 cup 100 percent white grape juice or grape juice, chilled

1. In a heat-proof bowl, stir the gelatin powder and boiling water until completely dissolved.

2. Drain canned fruit juice into a measuring cup, reserving fruit. Add enough grape juice to make 1¼ cups. Stir juice into the gelatin mixture and refrigerate for about 2 hours, or until slightly thickened.

3. Add the reserved fruit and stir gently to incorporate. Pour into a lightly greased 4- to 6-cup mold. Refrigerate for 3 to 4 hours, or until firm.

Fruity Morning Oatmeal

There are two schools of oatmeal eaters: those who like it plain and those who prefer it sweetened. If you are a member of the sweet camp, top with a bit of brown sugar.

2 servings

Prep Time:
15 minutes or less

Total Time:
15 minutes or less

Nutritional Information
Per Serving
Calories 270
Total Fat . . . . 5 g
Total Carbohydrate . . . . . . 46 g
Dietary Fiber . . . . 5 g
Sugars . . . . 17 g
Protein . . . . 13 g
Sodium . . . . 250 mg

1¾ **cups low-fat milk**
⅛ **teaspoon salt**
1 **cup old-fashioned rolled oats**
1 **apple, peeled, cored, and chopped**
1 **teaspoon light brown sugar, optional**

1. In a saucepan over medium-high heat, combine the milk and salt and bring to a boil. Reduce the heat to medium, stir in the oats and apple and cook, stirring occasionally, until thickened. Just before serving, sprinkle with brown sugar.

Oatmeal has many heart-healthy benefits. It is low in saturated fat and sodium and is full of iron, magnesium, and fiber. Oats can lower cholesterol levels because of their soluble-fiber content.

To adapt this recipe for people experiencing constipation, add dried fruit, such as raisins and dried cranberries, and leave the peel on the apple. You can also use a pear instead of the apple.

Adapted, with permission, from *The Great American Eat-Right Cookbook* (Atlanta, GA: American Cancer Society, 2007), 144.

Lemon–Egg Drop Soup

This simple, comforting meal comes together in less than half an hour. Enriched with eggs, this soup gets a touch of acidity from lemon juice—just enough to make it interesting. Add the juice of a third lemon if you are looking for stronger flavor. To add freshness, sprinkle with chopped fresh dill or Italian parsley just before serving.

Use leftover rice or buy packaged precooked rice. You can also use 1/3 cup instant rice, adding it to the broth after it boils. If you don't have cooked chicken on hand, you can also cook finely chopped raw chicken in the soup. Add 1 cup raw chicken with the rice and lemon juice and cook for 5 to 7 minutes, or until the chicken is cooked through.

6 servings

Prep Time:
15 minutes or less

Total Time:
30 minutes or less

Nutritional Information
Per Serving (about 1 cup)
Calories 80
Total Fat . . . . 2 g
Total Carbohydrate . . . . . . 10 g
Dietary Fiber . . . . 0 g
Sugars . . . . 1 g
Protein . . . . 5 g
Sodium . . . . 115 mg

6 cups reduced-sodium chicken broth
2 eggs
Juice of 2 lemons
1 cup cooked white rice
1 cup finely chopped cooked chicken, optional
Salt and freshly ground black pepper

1. In a large saucepan over high heat, bring the broth to a boil. Reduce the heat to a simmer.

2. Meanwhile, in a bowl, beat the eggs. Gradually, add 1 cup of the hot broth to the eggs a little at a time, beating constantly until the eggs are warmed through, but still liquid. You don't want the broth to cook the eggs, just to warm them through.

3. Over low heat, add the warm egg mixture back to the saucepan, stirring constantly. Add the lemon juice, rice, and chicken and cook for 3 to 5 minutes, or until heated through. Season with salt and pepper.

Mashed Potato–Chicken Patties

These little patties are perfect for sensitive stomachs and for those looking for an easy-to-eat small meal. Each bite provides comfort and sustenance. Cooked chicken breast adds lean protein while the potatoes provide carbohydrates.

This combination is also a great way to use up the leftovers from a chicken and potato dinner. Use a food processor to quickly grind the chicken.

8 servings

Prep Time:
15 minutes or less

Total Time:
30 minutes or less

Nutritional Information
Per Serving (about 1 patty)
Calories 90
Total Fat . . . . 3.5 g
Total Carbohydrate . . . . 8 g
Dietary Fiber . . . . 1 g
Sugars . . . . 1 g
Protein . . . . 6 g
Sodium . . . . 85 mg

If you don't have left-over mashed potatoes, make your own (see Mini Shepherd's Pies, page 29) or buy refrigerated premade mashed potatoes.

¼ cup all-purpose flour
Salt and freshly ground black pepper
1 egg
1 cup cooled mashed potatoes
1 cup (about 4 ounces) cooked chicken breast, ground or very finely chopped
1 tablespoon vegetable oil

1. On a plate, combine the flour and a sprinkle of salt and pepper.

2. In a bowl, beat the egg. Add the mashed potatoes and chicken. Form the mixture into 2-inch balls. Lightly dredge the balls in the flour. You may need to wet your hands after every 3 to 4 balls.

3. In a large, preferably nonstick, skillet over medium heat, add the oil. Add the balls and flatten into patties with a spatula (they should be about 2½ inches wide). Cook for 5 to 8 minutes per side, or until crispy and golden.

Chapter 3

Constipation can be caused by medication (especially pain and nausea medications), chemotherapy, and iron or calcium supplements. Dehydration, changes in your eating habits, and decreased physical activity may also contribute to constipation. Some chemotherapy regimens may intensify an existing problem with constipation, especially for the elderly and those who are eating low-fiber diets and not drinking enough liquid.

Constipation may affect your appetite—you may feel full more quickly than normal and excess gas may make you feel uncomfortable. To avoid discomfort, gradually increase your insoluble fiber intake. Insoluble fiber can be found in the skin and peel of vegetables and fruits and in whole grains. As you increase insoluble fiber, it is necessary to increase fluid intake to promote regularity. Try to drink at least 8 cups of liquid each day, unless otherwise directed by your health care team. Try water, warm prune juice, pasteurized fresh juices, and warm or hot fluids in the morning. Hot liquid in the morning can help to stimulate the bowels.

Inform your medical provider if you have not had a bowel movement in 2 to 3 days. Changes in your diet may not be powerful enough to correct constipation.

High-fiber foods such as these can help to soften the stool and ease constipation:

- Raw or cooked fruits and vegetables, with the skin and peel on (unless otherwise directed by your oncology team)

- Beans, peas, and nuts

- Dried fruit such as apricots, prunes, and raisins

- 100 percent bran or whole grain cereals, bread, popcorn, brown rice, and whole wheat pasta

If you are bloated or having problems with gas, avoid these gas-producing foods and beverages:

- Beans, peas, and nuts

- Vegetables such as broccoli, cauliflower, Brussels sprouts, cabbage, onions, garlic, cucumber, and bell pepper

- Carbonated beverages

- To lessen the amount of air you swallow while eating, try not to talk much at meals, do not use straws in drinks, and avoid chewing gum.

N	Nausea
D	Diarrhea
C	Constipation
SM	Sore Mouth and Difficulty Swallowing
TA	Taste Alterations
WL	Unintentional Weight Loss

These tips may be helpful in managing constipation:

• Avoid using extreme force or straining when trying to move your bowels.

• Try to eat and snack at the same times each day.

• Get as much light exercise as possible. Physical activity may help to stimulate the bowels. Ask your physician for guidelines.

• Use stool softeners, laxatives, or fiber supplements as instructed by your health care team. Adequate hydration is necessary for fiber supplements to work properly.

For more information about managing constipation,
contact the American Cancer Society at 800-227-2345
or visit our Web site at cancer.org.

Raisin-Bran Muffins

Fiber is an important part of a healthy diet, and these bran muffins are hearty without being heavy. Made with bran cereal, they take only a few minutes to whip up. You can add other dried fruit or nuts or omit the raisins.

12 muffins

Prep Time:
15 minutes or less

Total Time:
45 minutes or less

Nutritional Information
Per Serving (1 muffin)
Calories 195
Total Fat . . . . 6 g
Total Carbohydrate . . . . . . 35 g
Dietary Fiber . . . . 3 g
Sugars . . . . 19 g
Protein . . . . 4 g
Sodium . . . . 230 mg

If you don't have canola oil on hand, you can substitute any other vegetable oil.

½ **cup boiling water**
1½ **cups All-Bran or other 100 percent bran cereal**
1 **egg**
1 **cup buttermilk**
¼ **cup canola oil**
1¼ **cups all-purpose flour**
½ **cup (packed) light brown sugar**
1¼ **teaspoons baking soda**
½ **teaspoon ground cinnamon**
¼ **teaspoon salt**
1 **cup brown or golden raisins, or a mix**

1. Preheat the oven to 375 degrees. Coat a muffin tin with nonstick cooking spray or fill with paper liners.

2. In a heatproof bowl, pour the water over the cereal and stir to combine. Set aside.

3. In a separate bowl, beat the egg. Add the buttermilk and oil and stir to combine. Add the cereal mixture, flour, brown sugar, baking soda, cinnamon, and salt and stir until just combined. Add the raisins and stir gently to incorporate. Spoon the batter evenly into muffin cups.

4. Bake for 18 to 23 minutes, or until the tops just bounce back when touched. Leave in the tin for 5 minutes before transferring to a cooling rack.

Adapted, with permission, from *The Great American Eat-Right Cookbook* (Atlanta, GA: American Cancer Society, 2007), 137.

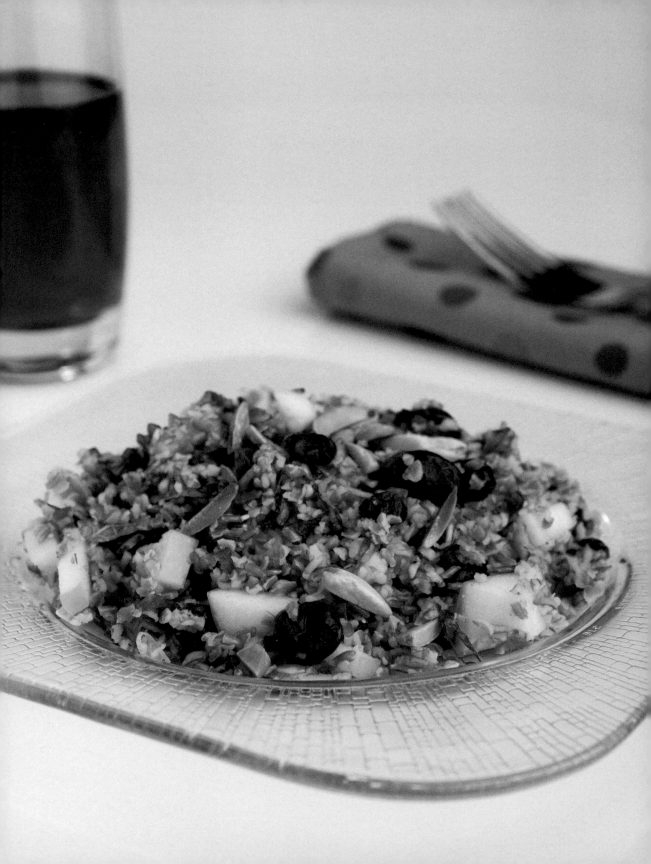

Bulgur Salad with Dried Fruit

Bulgur, also known as cracked wheat, is one of the most fiber-rich grains. Another plus—unlike other grains, it doesn't require a long cooking time. It only needs to be rehydrated in boiling water for about a half-hour.

Get all the other ingredients ready while the bulgur soaks. If you have some fresh Italian parsley on hand, chop ¼ cup of it and sprinkle over the salad before serving.

If you don't have the time or inclination to squeeze an orange, you can use a high-quality 100 percent orange juice that is freshly squeezed (not from concentrate). Be sure to buy juice that is pasteurized.

6 servings

Prep Time:
15 minutes or less

Total Time:
45 minutes or less
plus 1 or more hours
refrigeration

Nutritional Information
Per Serving (about ½ cup)
Calories 140
Total Fat . . . . 5 g
Total Carbohydrate . . . . . . 24 g
Dietary Fiber . . . . 4 g
Sugars . . . . 9 g
Protein . . . . 3 g
Sodium . . . . 7 mg

1 cup bulgur
1 cup boiling water
½ apple, chopped
¼ cup dried sweetened cranberries
¼ cup golden or brown raisins
2 scallions, thinly sliced
2 tablespoons chopped fresh mint
2 tablespoons olive oil
2 tablespoons fresh lemon juice
2 tablespoons fresh orange juice or high-quality store-bought
   orange juice
Salt and freshly ground black pepper
2 tablespoons slivered almonds, lightly toasted, optional

1. In a heatproof bowl, combine the bulgur and water and let stand for 30 minutes. If the mixture is absorbing the water too quickly, add 1 tablespoon or more water.

2. When the bulgur is tender, add the apple, cranberries, raisins, scallions, and mint. In a bowl, combine the olive oil, lemon juice, and orange juice. Add to the salad and stir gently to incorporate. Season with salt and pepper. Cover and refrigerate for at least 1 hour. Add the almonds just before serving.

Brown Rice and Chickpea Salad

This salad is an easy way to incorporate extra fiber, vitamins, and minerals into your diet. Unlike white rice, brown rice includes the bran and germ, making it a healthier and more fiber-rich choice. Unfortunately, its longer cooking time discourages many people from using it. To cut down on prep time, you can use packaged precooked rice or plan to prepare extra when making it for a side dish.

If the spices are too much for a sensitive stomach, omit them. If your taste buds need a little extra, add a pinch more.

12 servings

Prep Time:
30 minutes or less

Total time:
30 minutes or less

Nutritional Information
Per Serving (about ½ cup)
Calories 180
Total Fat . . . . 8 g
Total Carbohydrate . . . . . . 24 g
Dietary Fiber . . . . 4 g
Sugars . . . . 6 g
Protein . . . . 5 g
Sodium . . . . 140 mg

For added crunch and sweetness, add a chopped apple or pear to the dish before serving.

3 cups cooked brown rice
1 (15-ounce) can chickpeas, rinsed and drained
1 red bell pepper, seeded and chopped
½ cup golden raisins, brown raisins, or currants
¼ cup (packed) chopped fresh Italian parsley
¼ cup olive oil
2 tablespoons fresh lemon juice
½ teaspoon salt
¼ teaspoon ground cinnamon
¼ teaspoon ground cumin
½ teaspoon curry powder
½ cup slivered almonds, lightly toasted

1. In a bowl, combine the rice and chickpeas. Add the red pepper, raisins, and parsley and stir to combine.

2. In a separate bowl, combine the oil, lemon juice, salt, cinnamon, cumin, and curry powder. Add to the salad and stir gently to combine. Add the almonds just before serving.

Fruity Bran Purée

A couple of spoonfuls of this combination may help promote regularity. Spread on toast or stir into hot cereal or yogurt. The mixture will keep for up to one week when covered and refrigerated.

5 servings

Prep Time:
15 minutes or less

Total Time:
15 minutes or less

Nutritional Information
Per Serving (2 tablespoons)
Calories 60
Total Fat . . . . 0 g
Total Carbohydrate . . . . . . 14 g
Dietary Fiber . . . . 2 g
Sugars . . . . 10 g
Protein . . . . 1 g
Sodium . . . . 30 mg

½ **cup applesauce**
½ **cup stewed prunes, pits removed**
½ **cup wheat bran flakes**

1. In a blender, combine the applesauce, prunes, and bran flakes and blend until smooth.

Adapted, with permission, from *Eating Well, Staying Well During and After Cancer* (Atlanta, GA: American Cancer Society, 2004), 216.

Honey-Yogurt Parfait with Dried Fruit and Granola

Layering yogurt with fruit and crunchy granola is a great way to maximize textures in a healthful breakfast or snack. Fresh fruit, such as berries, can be substituted for dried fruit if you prefer.

Greek yogurt (such as the Fage brand) is strained, so it's extra thick and creamy. It is also much higher in protein than regular yogurt. Sweetening it to taste with honey gives it added lushness with less sugar than many presweetened yogurts.

The parfait looks enticing served in a goblet, wine glass, or wide-bottomed clear tumbler. With a narrow glass, you'll be able to get two layers; if your glass or bowl is wider, just one should do it. If your appetite is up to it, double the layers.

1 serving

Prep Time:
15 minutes or less

Total Time:
15 minutes or less

**Nutritional Information
Per Serving**
Calories 335
Total Fat . . . . 5 g
Total Carbohydrate . . . . . . 60 g
Dietary Fiber . . . . 4 g
Sugars . . . . 43 g
Protein . . . . 14 g
Sodium . . . . 50 mg

½ **cup plain nonfat or low-fat yogurt, preferably Greek yogurt**
2 teaspoons honey
¼ **cup mixed chopped dried fruit, including raisins, apricots, and sweetened cranberries**
¼ **cup granola**

1. In a bowl, combine the yogurt and honey. Transfer to a serving glass and layer with dried fruit and granola.

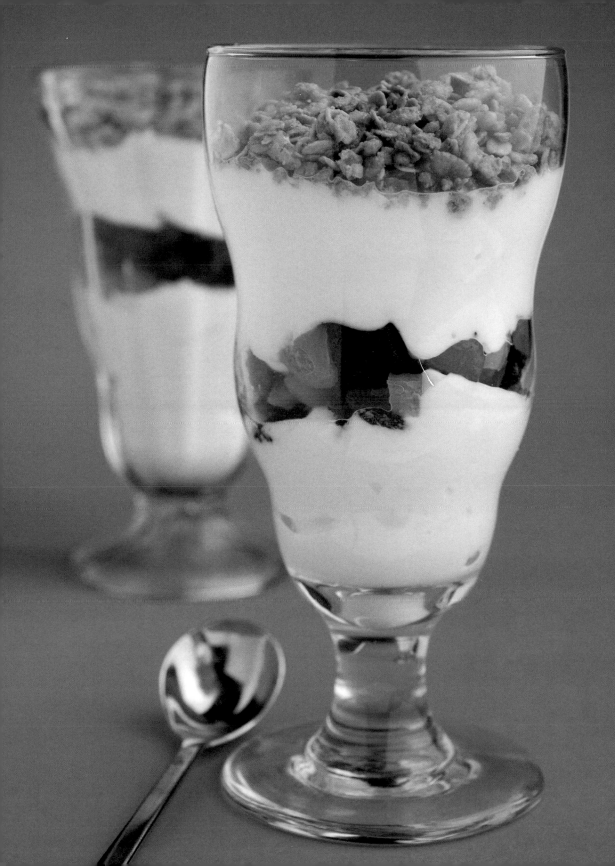

Spinach and Brown Rice Pie

This tasty casserole has the flavors of the Greek dish spanakopita, but with less fat and less work. It can be served as a vegetarian entrée or as a side dish to a simple protein-based meal. Its Mediterranean flavors are a perfect match for grilled chicken or fish.

This recipe is a great way to use up leftover rice. To save time, you can also use precooked packaged or quick-cooking rice.

8 to 10 servings

Prep Time:
15 minutes or less

Total Time:
45 minutes or less

Nutritional Information
Per Serving
Calories 185
Total Fat . . . . 8 g
Total Carbohydrate . . . . . . 20 g
Dietary Fiber . . . . 3 g
Sugars . . . . 4 g
Protein . . . . 11 g
Sodium . . . . 260 mg

2 eggs
2 (10-ounce) packages frozen chopped spinach, thawed, squeezed of excess liquid, and patted dry
3 scallions, thinly sliced
2 cups cooked brown rice or 1 (8.8-ounce) package precooked brown rice
½ cup crumbled feta cheese
½ cup grated Parmesan cheese
Salt and freshly ground black pepper
3 tablespoons butter
3 tablespoons all-purpose flour
1²⁄₃ cups low-fat milk

1. Preheat the oven to 350 degrees. Coat a pie plate with nonstick cooking spray.

2. In a large bowl, beat the eggs. Add the spinach, scallions, rice, feta, and Parmesan cheese and stir well to combine. Sprinkle with salt and pepper.

3. In a saucepan over low heat, melt the butter. Add the flour and cook until fully incorporated, stirring constantly. Gradually add the milk and bring to a light simmer for 3 to 5 minutes, or until thickened, stirring constantly. Pour the milk mixture over the spinach and stir well to combine. Transfer to the pie plate.

4. Bake for 25 to 30 minutes, or until golden. Let cool for 5 minutes before serving.

Black Bean Cakes

This high-fiber vegetarian dish is flavorful enough to please the whole family. To speed the prep time, chop the vegetables individually in the food processor before adding them to the skillet. Another time-saving tip is to prepare quick-cooking barley or make barley the night before as a side dish and reserve ¹/₂ cup to use here.

10 servings

Prep Time:
30 minutes or less

Total Time:
30 minutes or less

Nutritional Information
Per Serving
(about 2 miniature cakes)
Calories 115
Total Fat . . . . 4.5 g
Total Carbohydrate . . . . . . 15 g
Dietary Fiber . . . . 3 g
Sugars . . . . 2 g
Protein . . . . 5 g
Sodium . . . . 220 mg

Omit the hot sauce
and onion if you have
a sore mouth or throat.
Consider serving with
salsa if mouth soreness
is not a problem.

2 tablespoons olive oil or vegetable oil, divided
1 carrot, finely chopped
¹/₂ red bell pepper, seeded and finely chopped
¹/₂ onion, finely chopped
2 eggs
1 (15-ounce) can black beans, rinsed and drained
1 (4-ounce) can chopped green chiles, undrained
¹/₂ cup seasoned bread crumbs
¹/₂ cup cooked barley
1 tablespoon grated Parmesan cheese
¹/₄ teaspoon garlic salt
Dash hot sauce, or to taste

1. In a medium skillet over medium-high heat, add 1 tablespoon of the oil. Sauté the carrot, red pepper, and onion for 5 to 8 minutes, or until tender.

2. Meanwhile, in a bowl, beat the eggs. Add the beans and mash coarsely with a fork or potato masher. Add the chiles, bread crumbs, barley, Parmesan cheese, garlic salt, and hot sauce. Add the sautéed vegetables and stir gently to incorporate. Form the mixture into 1½-inch balls.

3. In a large, preferably nonstick, skillet over medium heat, add the remaining tablespoon of oil. Add the balls and flatten into cakes with a spatula (they should be about 2 inches wide). Cook for 2 to 5 minutes per side or until crispy and brown (you may need to do this step in two or more batches, depending on the size of your skillet).

Adapted, with permission, from *Celebrate! Healthy Entertaining for Any Occasion* (Atlanta, GA: American Cancer Society, 2001), 9.

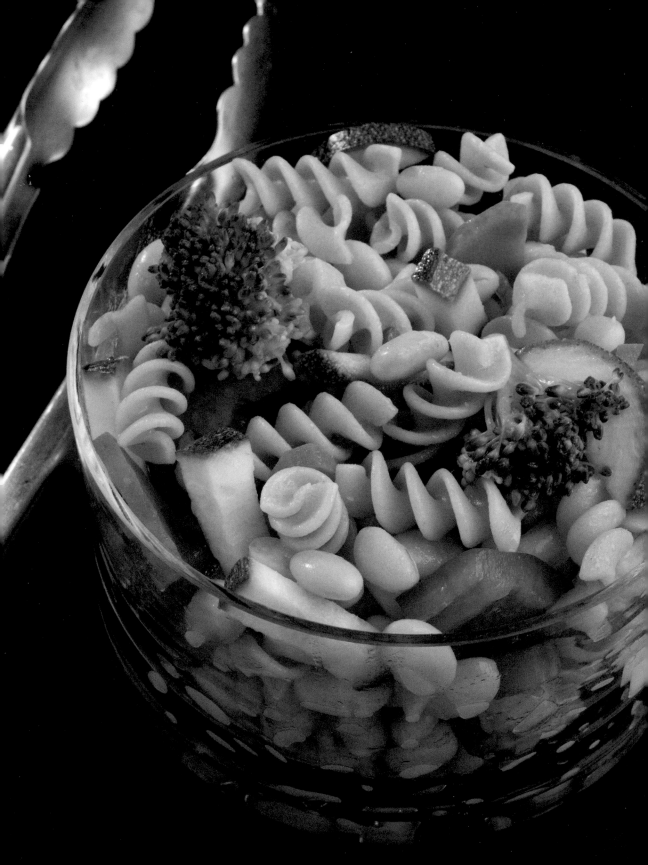

Minestrone Salad

This make-ahead dish includes lots of good-for-you, fiber-rich ingredients, including whole wheat pasta, beans, broccoli, and other vegetables. If the broccoli upsets your stomach, you can leave it out and use more of the other vegetables. If you like broccoli, feel free to add another cup.

For a nice presentation, serve on lettuce leaves with tomato slices.

13 servings

Prep Time:
30 minutes or less

Total Time:
30 minutes or less

Nutritional Information
Per Serving (about 1 cup)
Calories 180
Total Fat . . . . 6 g
Total Carbohydrate . . . . . . 29 g
Dietary Fiber . . . . 5 g
Sugars . . . . 4 g
Protein . . . . 6 g
Sodium . . . . 350 mg

12 ounces whole wheat elbow, fusilli, or other shaped pasta
2 to 3 cups small broccoli florets
1 (15-ounce) can Great Northern beans, rinsed and drained
4 scallions, white and green parts, thinly sliced
2 carrots, sliced in half lengthwise and sliced
1 zucchini, cut into rounds and sliced into strips
1 red or green bell pepper, seeded and chopped
1 to 1½ cups regular or reduced-fat Italian salad dressing
Salt and freshly ground black pepper

1. Prepare the pasta according to package directions. During the last 3 minutes of cooking, add the broccoli to the pot. After draining, rinse with cold water.

2. Meanwhile, in a large bowl, combine the beans, scallions, carrots, zucchini, and bell pepper. Add the drained pasta mixture and 1 cup of the salad dressing and stir gently to incorporate. Add more dressing if needed. Season with salt and pepper.

Adapted, with permission, from *The American Cancer Society's Healthy Eating Cookbook, Third Edition* (Atlanta, GA: American Cancer Society, 2005), 58.

Fiber-Filled Trail Mix

"Trail mixes" can provide calories when you need to eat but can't face a "traditional" meal. This mix is an easy and filling snack that also provides fiber and protein through a combination of dried fruits, seeds, and nuts.

11 servings

Prep Time:
15 minutes or less

Total Time:
15 minutes or less

2 cups air-popped popcorn

1 cup high-fiber cereal, such as Mini Wheats, Crunchy Corn Bran, Wheat Chex, or granola

½ cup roasted salted peanuts or almonds

½ cup dried apricots

½ cup dried cherries or raisins

½ cup dried sweetened cranberries

½ cup sunflower seeds

Nutritional Information
Per Serving (about ½ cup)
Calories 150
Total Fat . . . . 6 g
Total Carbohydrate . . . . . . 23 g
Dietary Fiber . . . . 3 g
Sugars . . . . 14 g
Protein . . . . 4 g
Sodium . . . . 55 mg

1. In a container with an airtight lid, combine the popcorn, cereal, peanuts, apricots, cherries, cranberries, and sunflower seeds.

This is a good snack to keep in your car or take to treatment. If you need to gain weight, increase the serving size.

Fruit Smoothie

This nondairy drink offers a burst of fruity flavor. For a frosty drink, use frozen berries instead of fresh. Instead of buying individual bags of frozen berries, you can use a bag of mixed berries or choose another fruit you prefer. For a less acidic drink, use apple or pomegranate juice instead of orange juice.

Add protein powder for extra calories and protein. You can also add 1 cup or a 6-ounce container of plain, vanilla, or fruit yogurt for extra protein.

3 servings

Prep Time:
15 minutes or less

Total Time:
15 minutes or less

Nutritional Information
Per Serving (about ³/₄ cup)
Calories 100
Total Fat . . . . 1 g
Total Carbohydrate . . . . . . 24 g
Dietary Fiber . . . . 4 g
Sugars . . . . 18 g
Protein . . . . 1 g
Sodium . . . . 5 mg

¹/₂ **cup fresh or frozen blueberries**
¹/₂ **cup fresh or frozen strawberries, hulled if fresh**
¹/₂ **cup fresh or frozen blackberries**
¹/₂ **cup fresh or frozen raspberries**
1 ¹/₂ **cups apple juice, orange juice, or other fruit juice**

1. In a blender, combine the blueberries, strawberries, blackberries, raspberries, and juice and blend until smooth.

Adapted, with permission, from *Eating Well, Staying Well During and After Cancer* (Atlanta, GA: American Cancer Society, 2004), 213.

Blueberry-Peach Crisp

A baked crisp is a tasty way to enjoy fruit in a slightly sweetened form. With frozen peaches and blueberries readily available, you can enjoy this combination of fruits all year. You can substitute fresh seasonal fruit—just cut back the covered baking time by about 15 minutes.

If you don't have a food processor, use a pastry blender or fork to cut in the butter until crumbly.

If you're trying to gain weight, top with whipped cream or ice cream.

6 servings

Prep Time:
15 minutes or less

Total Time:
1 hour or less

Nutritional Information
Per Serving

Calories 305
Total Fat . . . . 9 g
Total Carbohydrate . . . . . . 56 g
Dietary Fiber . . . . 4 g
Sugars . . . . 37 g
Protein . . . . 3 g
Sodium . . . . 65 mg

For a stronger flavor, add another teaspoon of cinnamon to the fruit mixture.

3 cups frozen sliced peaches
2 cups frozen blueberries
¼ cup granulated sugar
2 tablespoons plus ½ cup all-purpose flour, divided
½ cup quick-cooking oats
½ cup (packed) light brown sugar
1 teaspoon ground cinnamon
4 tablespoons butter, cut into pieces

1. Preheat the oven to 350 degrees.

2. In an 8-by-8-inch baking pan, combine the peaches and blueberries. In a bowl, combine sugar and 2 tablespoons of the flour. Add to fruit, stirring well to combine.

3. In a food processor, combine the remaining ½ cup flour, oats, brown sugar, and cinnamon and pulse briefly to combine. Add the butter and process until mixture is moist throughout and begins to clump together. Sprinkle over fruit and cover tightly with foil.

4. Bake for 30 minutes. Remove the foil and bake for an additional 15 minutes, or until fruit is tender and mixture is bubbly. Let cool for 5 to 10 minutes before serving.

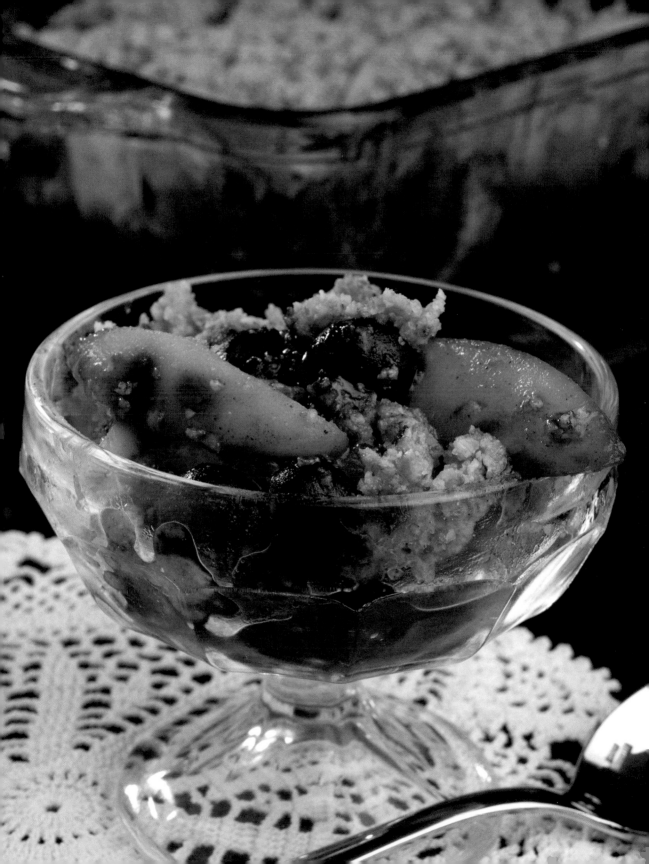

Rosemary–White Bean Soup

Using canned beans in this recipe allows you to skip the step of soaking beans overnight, making this soup a perfect last-minute "what's in the cupboard" meal.

Use caution when puréeing a hot soup. Cool slightly before puréeing and avoid filling the blender or food processor more than three-quarters full.

If the soup is too thick for your liking, dilute with broth or water.

6 servings

Prep Time:
15 minutes or less

Total Time:
45 minutes or less

Nutritional Information
Per Serving (about 1 cup)
Calories 215
Total Fat . . . . 3 g
Total Carbohydrate . . . . . . 36 g
Dietary Fiber . . . . 8 g
Sugars . . . . 5 g
Protein . . . . 12 g
Sodium . . . . 600 mg

1 tablespoon vegetable oil
1 onion, chopped
1 carrot, chopped
1 celery stalk, chopped
2 garlic cloves, finely chopped
4 cups reduced-sodium chicken broth or vegetable broth
3 (15-ounce) cans navy or Great Northern beans, rinsed and drained
1 (4-inch) sprig fresh rosemary
Salt and freshly ground black pepper

1. In a stockpot over medium-high heat, add the oil. Sauté the onion, carrot, and celery for 5 to 7 minutes, or until softened. Add the garlic and sauté for 1 to 2 minutes. Add the broth and beans and stir to combine. Bring to a boil. Reduce the heat, add the rosemary, and simmer for 20 to 25 minutes, stirring occasionally. Cool slightly and remove the rosemary.

2. Transfer to a blender or food processor and purée (you may need to do this step in two or more batches). Season with salt and pepper.

Hummus

Eating hummus with whole wheat pita and baby carrots or broccoli is a quick way to get fiber, calories, and protein.

Tahini is a high-fat paste made from ground sesame seeds. The oil will separate from the paste, so make sure to stir well before using. Look for tahini in the international food aisle of your supermarket.

If desired, sprinkle the hummus with chopped fresh Italian parsley.

7 servings

Prep Time:
15 minutes or less

Total Time:
15 minutes or less

Nutritional Information
Per Serving (about ¼ cup)
Calories 145
Total Fat . . . . 10 g
Total Carbohydrate . . . . . . 12 g
Dietary Fiber . . . . 4 g
Sugars . . . . 2 g
Protein . . . . 5 g
Sodium . . . . 240 mg

Chickpeas are also known as garbanzo beans and are a good source of fiber.

2 garlic cloves
1 (15-ounce) can chickpeas, rinsed and drained
¼ cup tahini
3 tablespoons fresh lemon juice, or to taste
3 tablespoons hot water
2 tablespoons olive oil
1 teaspoon ground cumin, or to taste
½ teaspoon salt, or to taste

1. In a food processor, with the motor running, drop in the garlic and purée. Stop the machine, add the chickpeas, tahini, lemon juice, water, oil, cumin, and salt, and process until smooth. Taste and add more lemon juice, cumin, or salt, if needed.

Adapted, with permission, from *The American Cancer Society's Healthy Eating Cookbook, Third Edition* (Atlanta, GA: American Cancer Society, 2005), 17.

Blueberry-Banana-Oatmeal Smoothie

Blueberries are a good source of fiber and naturally occurring antioxidants. If you are lactose intolerant or dairy products upset your stomach, you can substitute lactose-free milk for the low-fat milk.

2 servings

Prep Time:
15 minutes or less

Total Time:
15 minutes or less

Nutritional Information
Per Serving (about 1 cup)
Calories 250
Total Fat . . . . 2 g
Total Carbohydrate . . . . . . 54 g
Dietary Fiber . . . . 4 g
Sugars . . . . 40 g
Protein . . . . 6 g
Sodium . . . . 70 mg

The amount of oats in this recipe can be increased. Because the oats affect the texture, however, start with 1 tablespoon and add more as you develop a taste for it.

1 tablespoon old-fashioned rolled oats
1 ripe banana, broken into pieces
1 cup frozen blueberries, raspberries, or other fruit
1 (6-ounce) container blueberry, strawberry, or vanilla low-fat yogurt
½ cup low-fat milk or lactose-free milk
1 to 2 tablespoons honey
Pinch ground cinnamon

1. In a blender, purée the oats. Add the banana, blueberries, yogurt, milk, 1 tablespoon of the honey, and cinnamon and blend until smooth. Taste and add the remaining tablespoon of honey if necessary.

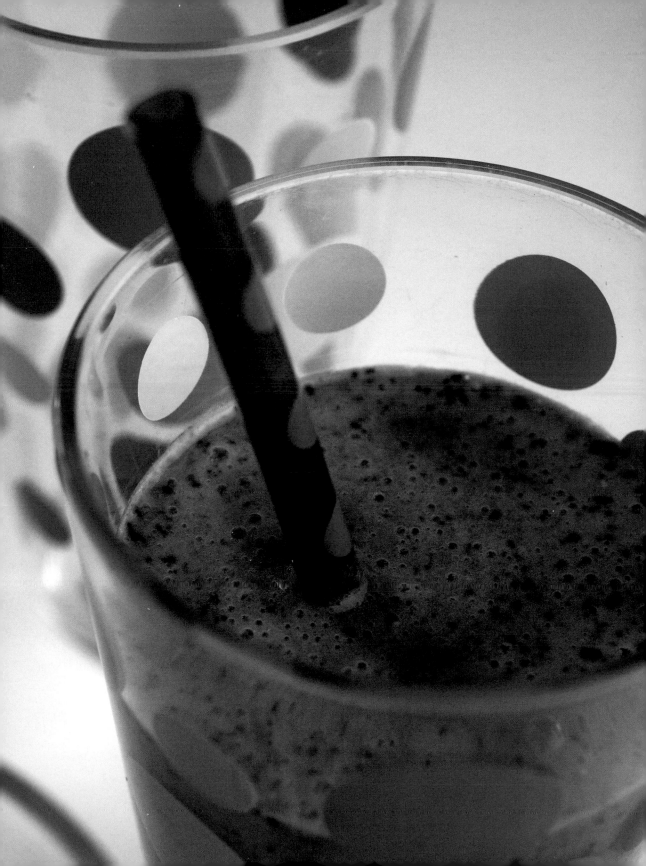

Tuscan White Bean Salad

This easy recipe makes a flavorful side dish, sandwich filling, or an elegant appetizer. Serve as is, tuck inside soft pita bread, or mash the mixture slightly and mound on top of toasted Italian bread slices for crostini.

Toss the ingredients together about 30 minutes before serving so the salad can chill in the refrigerator.

11 servings

Prep Time:
30 minutes or less

Total Time:
1 hour or less
including refrigeration

Nutritional Information
Per Serving (about ½ cup)
Calories 110
Total Fat . . . . 4.5 g
Total Carbohydrate . . . . . . 13 g
Dietary Fiber . . . . 3 g
Sugars . . . . 2 g
Protein . . . . 5 g
Sodium . . . . 125 mg

1 teaspoon plus 2 tablespoons olive oil, divided
1 garlic clove, finely chopped
1 teaspoon dried oregano
2 to 3 tablespoons cider vinegar
2 (15-ounce) cans cannellini beans or Great Northern beans, rinsed and drained
4 plum tomatoes, chopped
½ Vidalia or other sweet onion, finely chopped
½ cup crumbled feta cheese
½ cup chopped fresh Italian parsley
Salt and freshly ground black pepper

1. In a nonstick skillet over medium-high heat, add 1 teaspoon of the oil. Sauté the garlic and oregano for 30 seconds to 1 minute, or until aromatic. Remove from heat and stir in 2 tablespoons of the vinegar.

2. In a large bowl, combine the beans, tomatoes, onion, feta, and parsley. Add the remaining 2 tablespoons oil and the vinegar mixture and stir gently to incorporate. Taste and add more vinegar if necessary. Season with salt and pepper. Cover and refrigerate for at least 30 minutes.

Adapted, with permission, from *Celebrate! Healthy Entertaining for Any Occasion* (Atlanta, GA: American Cancer Society, 2001), 67.

Chapter 4

SORE MOUTH AND DIFFICULTY SWALLOWING

Cancer or cancer treatment can cause some individuals to develop mouth ulcers or a sore mouth or throat. Certain chemotherapy agents and radiation therapy to the head and neck area and even to the chest can cause these symptoms. Be sure your physician knows early on about any mouth problems so that appropriate treatment can be prescribed. Your physician may actually prescribe techniques and therapies to try to prevent mouth sores from occurring.

Inflammation and mouth sores can make eating painful, and your favorite foods may irritate your mouth. If you are having severe pain that interferes with eating, ask your doctor about medication to relieve pain. Some medicines can be swished in the mouth before meals, and there are others that can be dabbed on the painful areas with a cotton swab before eating.

Trouble swallowing can also be a problematic side effect. This can lead to loss of appetite, weight loss, and dehydration. If you are having trouble swallowing, your doctor may be able to prescribe a local anesthetic or pain reliever to coat your throat. Do not force yourself to eat if you cannot swallow. Follow your health care team's instructions for special eating techniques.

If you are experiencing mouth sores or trouble swallowing, soft or semisoft, bland, room-temperature foods will probably be easier to eat and swallow.

These suggestions may be helpful for managing sore mouth and difficulty swallowing:

- Eat soft foods such as cream soups, cheeses, mashed potatoes, yogurt, eggs, custards, puddings, cooked cereals, ice cream, and casseroles.

- Moisten dry foods with broth, gravy, or sauces.

- Blend or purée foods in a blender to make them easier to swallow. Add enough liquid (broth, juice, or milk) to achieve the desired consistency.

- Avoid tart, acidic, or salty foods and drinks such as citrus fruits (grapefruit, orange, lemon, and lime), pickled and vinegar-based foods, and tomato-based foods and drinks.

- Avoid rough-textured foods, such as dry toast, crackers, pretzels, granola, raw fruits and vegetables, or fried or baked foods with rough exteriors.

- Choose lukewarm or cool foods. Very hot food may cause discomfort. Some people find icy foods to be soothing.

N	Nausea
D	Diarrhea
C	Constipation
SM	Sore Mouth and Difficulty Swallowing
TA	Taste Alterations
WL	Unintentional Weight Loss

- Eat small, frequent meals and snacks. It is usually easier to eat smaller portions more frequently.

If you are having trouble swallowing, thick liquids may be more easily tolerated than thin. There are several ways to thicken food and liquids:

- Mix 1 tablespoon of unflavored gelatin in 2 cups of liquid until dissolved and pour over cakes, cookies, crackers, sandwiches, puréed fruits, and other cold foods. Allow food to sit until firm.

- Use tapioca, flour, and cornstarch to thicken liquids. Note that these substances must be cooked.

- Use puréed vegetables and instant potatoes in soups.

- Use baby rice cereal to make very thick liquids.

- You can also use commercial thickeners (found at your local pharmacy) to adjust the thickness of a food or liquid. Follow label instructions.

Call your health care team if you cough or choke routinely while eating, especially if you develop a fever afterward. This could be a sign that you are having swallowing problems.

For more information about managing mouth sores or trouble swallowing, contact the American Cancer Society at 800-227-2345 or visit our Web site at cancer.org.

Chilled Cucumber and Yogurt Soup

This cold soup offers subtle flavors in a refreshing way, especially if your mouth is sensitive to heat. To seed the cucumber, simply slice in half lengthwise and use a spoon to scoop out the seeds from the middle.

6 servings

Prep Time:
15 minutes or less

Total Time:
15 minutes or less
plus 2 or more hours
refrigeration

**Nutritional Information
Per Serving (about 1 cup)**
Calories 80
Total Fat . . . . 2.5 g
Total Carbohydrate . . . . . . 11 g
Dietary Fiber . . . . 1 g
Sugars . . . . 9 g
Protein . . . . 5 g
Sodium . . . . 830 mg

> This low-fat soup is also good for weight reduction.
>
> If garlic is bothersome, you can leave it out.

1 large garlic clove

2 tablespoons fresh dill, thick stems removed

3 medium cucumbers, peeled, seeded, and coarsely chopped (about 4 cups)

2 cups plain nonfat yogurt or Greek yogurt

2 cups water

1 tablespoon olive oil

1 tablespoon honey

2 teaspoons salt

1 teaspoon ground black pepper

1. In a food processor, with the motor running, drop in the garlic and dill and purée. Stop the machine, add the cucumbers, and pulse until finely chopped. Add the yogurt, water, oil, honey, salt, and pepper and pulse 2 or 3 times just to combine. Do not overprocess.

2. Transfer to a large bowl. Cover and refrigerate for at least 2 hours. If the soup thickens too much, dilute with ice cubes.

Ribollita

This peasant-style vegetable soup originated when Italian cooks were looking for ways to stretch out their minestrone soup and added their leftover bread.

For some, this soup is best enjoyed when the bread has just been added and still has some firmness. Others like it even better when the bread absorbs the liquid and the ribollita takes on a thick porridge-like consistency. Because the bread absorbs so much broth, if you're not eating all the soup at once, only add bread to the portion you're planning to serve.

For added flavor, top each serving with Parmesan cheese.

10 servings

Prep Time:
15 minutes or less

Total Time:
1 hour or less

Nutritional Information
Per Serving (about 1 cup)
Calories 125
Total Fat . . . . 3 g
Total Carbohydrate . . . . . . 19 g
Dietary Fiber . . . . 3 g
Sugars . . . . 3 g
Protein . . . . 6 g
Sodium . . . . 750 mg

You can freeze half the soup to have later—just wait to add the bread until you're ready to serve.

Dirt can get trapped in the leek, so be sure to wash well before using.

This recipe is good for people who are having swallowing problems. If you have mouth sores, you may need to omit the diced tomatoes.

2 tablespoons olive oil
1 leek, white part only, thinly sliced or 1 small onion, chopped
2 garlic cloves, finely chopped
1 carrot, finely chopped
1 celery stalk, finely chopped
½ head Savoy cabbage, sliced thinly, optional
6 cups reduced-sodium chicken broth
1 (14.5-ounce) can diced tomatoes
1 (15-ounce) can cannellini or small white beans, rinsed and drained
1 teaspoon salt
½ teaspoon ground black pepper
2 cups stale crusty sourdough, French, or Italian bread, cut into 1-inch pieces
¼ cup fresh basil, coarsely chopped
Grated Parmesan cheese, optional

1. In a stockpot over medium-high heat, add the oil. Sauté the leek for 5 minutes. Add the garlic, carrot, and celery and sauté for 5 to 8 minutes, or until softened. Add the cabbage and sauté for 2 to 3 minutes. Add the broth and tomatoes and stir to combine. Bring to a boil. Add the beans, salt, and pepper and stir to combine. Reduce the heat and simmer for 20 minutes, stirring occasionally.

2. Add the bread and basil and cook for 3 to 5 minutes. Serve with Parmesan cheese.

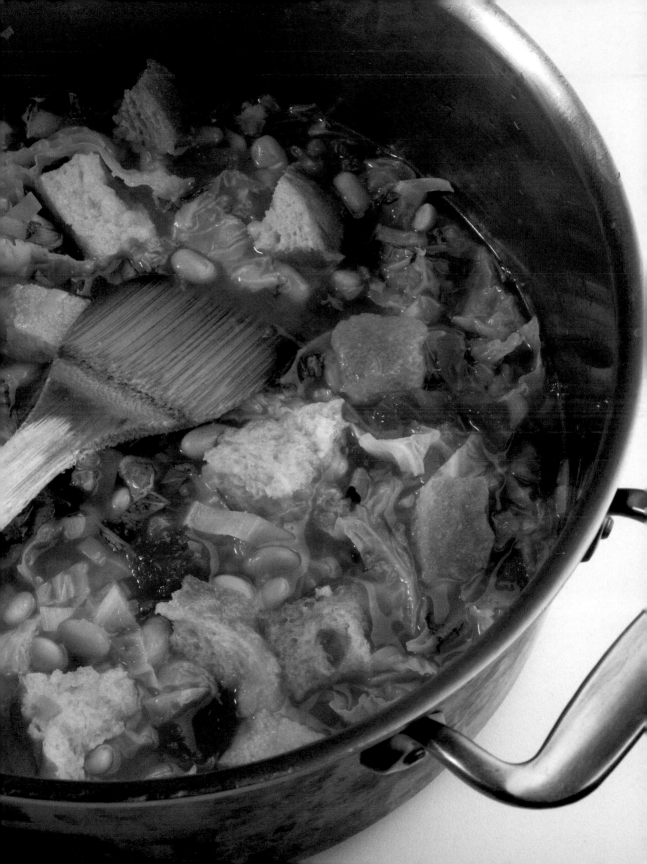

Frosty Coffee Shake

When your mouth is sensitive to heat but you still crave that coffee pick-me-up, try this frosty coffeehouse-style beverage. Freezing coffee in ice cube trays allows you to get the chill you want without diluting the flavor with ice. A healthy dose of milk mellows the drink and adds calcium.

For a mocha treat, add chocolate syrup to taste. If the coffee flavor is too strong, add ice cubes.

1 serving

Prep Time:
15 minutes or less

Total Time:
15 minutes or less
plus 3 or more hours
freezing

**Nutritional Information
Per Serving**
Calories 150
Total Fat . . . . 1 g
Total Carbohydrate . . . . . . 31 g
Dietary Fiber . . . . 0 g
Sugars . . . . 31 g
Protein . . . . 4 g
Sodium . . . . 60 mg

If you are trying to gain weight, use whole milk.

Freeze cooled coffee in ice cube trays and then transfer the frozen coffee cubes to a zip-top bag to have them ready when you need them. Forgot to measure? A cup is about 9 to 12 regular-sized ice cubes. To make iced coffee or for a weaker drink, try chilled coffee and ice.

1 cup strong regular or decaffeinated coffee, frozen in ice cube trays
½ cup low-fat or whole milk
2 tablespoons granulated sugar

1. In a blender, combine the coffee ice cubes, milk, and sugar and blend until smooth.

Strawberry Frozen Yogurt Popsicles

These refreshing snacks provide all the nutrients of a smoothie, but in solid lickable form. If your Popsicle mold doesn't come with individual handles, freeze the mixture until partially set, insert a wooden stick into each mold, and then freeze until solid. You can also use small paper cups if you don't have a Popsicle mold.

4 servings

Prep Time:
15 minutes or less

Total Time:
**15 minutes or less
plus 3 or more hours
freezing**

**Nutritional Information
Per Serving**
Calories 95
Total Fat . . . . 1 g
Total Carbohydrate . . . . . . 20 g
Dietary Fiber . . . . 1 g
Sugars . . . . 14 g
Protein . . . . 2 g
Sodium . . . . 35 mg

Adding corn syrup helps prevent ice crystals from forming, keeping the texture of the Popsicles smooth.

1 cup strawberry or other flavored low-fat yogurt
1½ cups (about 12) fresh or frozen strawberries, hulled if fresh, or other fruit, divided
1 tablespoon light corn syrup
1 teaspoon fresh lemon juice

1. In a food processor, combine the yogurt, 1 cup of the strawberries, corn syrup, and lemon juice and process until smooth. Add the remaining ¹/₂ cup berries and pulse until fruit is mostly puréed but some small pieces of fruit remain. Pour into four (¹/₂-cup) Popsicle molds and insert tops. Freeze until solid, at least 3 hours.

2. To remove the pops from the molds, run the outside of the mold under hot water. The ice pop should loosen and pull out.

Roasted Cauliflower Soup

This creamy, mild soup requires almost no labor. The main flavoring comes simply from the caramelization of the roasted cauliflower. A hint of cream adds lushness.

5 servings

Prep Time:
15 minutes or less

Total Time:
1 hour or less

Nutritional Information
Per Serving (about 1 cup)
Calories 135
Total Fat . . . . 12 g
Total Carbohydrate . . . . 5 g
Dietary Fiber . . . . 2 g
Sugars . . . . 2 g
Protein . . . . 4 g
Sodium . . . . 380 mg

For stronger flavor, add two to three minced garlic cloves to the cauliflower before roasting. Another option is to sprinkle cauliflower with 1 teaspoon fresh thyme leaves and/or 2 tablespoons freshly grated Parmesan cheese during the last 5 to 10 minutes of roasting.

To increase calories, use up to 1 cup heavy cream. If watching calories, omit cream altogether or substitute 1/2 cup low-fat milk.

This recipe may not be suitable if you are experiencing gas.

1 large (about 2 pounds) head cauliflower, cut into large florets
1 to 2 tablespoons olive oil
Salt and freshly ground black pepper
3½ to 4 cups reduced-sodium chicken broth or vegetable broth, heated
½ to 1 cup heavy cream

1. Preheat the oven to 425 degrees.

2. On a foil-lined, rimmed baking sheet, drizzle cauliflower with oil and toss to coat. Sprinkle with salt and pepper. Roast for 25 to 35 minutes, or until very tender and slightly charred, tossing every 10 minutes.

3. Transfer to a blender and add 3½ cups of the warmed broth and 1/2 cup of the cream. Blend until smooth, adding more broth or cream to achieve desired consistency. (You may need to do this step in batches or transfer some of the mixture to a large bowl before adding all the liquid.)

Peanut Butter–Banana Shake

Peanut butter and banana have always been a winning combo, both for taste and nutritional value. Peanut butter provides protein and unsaturated fat and bananas are full of potassium, both good things to incorporate into your diet if you're having trouble eating.

Chocolate syrup or honey adds a hint of sweetness to this mild shake.

2 servings

Prep Time:
15 minutes or less

Total Time:
15 minutes or less

Nutritional Information
Per Serving (about 1 cup)
Calories 350
Total Fat . . . . 19 g
Total Carbohydrate . . . . . . 34 g
Dietary Fiber . . . . 3 g
Sugars . . . . 22 g
Protein . . . . 12 g
Sodium . . . . 70 mg

The unused banana half can be wrapped in foil or plastic wrap and frozen for later use.

4 to 6 ice cubes
1 cup low-fat milk
½ large ripe banana, broken into pieces
¼ cup creamy all-natural or regular peanut butter
2 tablespoons chocolate syrup or honey

1. In a blender, crush 4 ice cubes. Add the milk, banana, peanut butter, and chocolate syrup and blend until smooth. For a colder shake, add the remaining ice cubes and blend until combined.

Pumpkin Shake

This frosty shake with an unexpected ingredient—pumpkin purée—will be a hit with all ages and all members of the family, but it is also great for a sore mouth. If you have pumpkin pie spice on hand, substitute 1 teaspoon for the spices listed below. To add more calories, substitute premium vanilla ice cream for the yogurt.

1 serving

Prep Time:
15 minutes or less

Total Time:
15 minutes or less

**Nutritional Information
Per Serving**
Calories 300
Total Fat . . . . 4.5 g
Total Carbohydrate . . . . . . 61 g
Dietary Fiber . . . . 4 g
Sugars . . . . 47 g
Protein . . . . 7 g
Sodium . . . . 100 mg

> Pumpkin contains beta carotene, vitamin A, and fiber.
>
> Use leftover pumpkin purée for the Pumpkin-Ginger Mini Muffins (page 16) or Pumpkin Custard (page 68).

2 to 3 ice cubes
½ cup canned pumpkin purée
½ cup low-fat milk
½ cup vanilla reduced-fat frozen yogurt
2 tablespoons maple syrup
¼ teaspoon ground cinnamon
Pinch ground nutmeg
Pinch ground allspice
Pinch ground ginger

1. In a blender, crush 2 ice cubes. Add the pumpkin, milk, frozen yogurt, maple syrup, cinnamon, nutmeg, allspice, and ginger and blend until smooth. For a colder shake, add the remaining ice cube and blend until combined.

Potato Soup

This mild soup is easy on the stomach and the mouth. The soup thickens when chilled and may need to be thinned with additional chicken broth or milk before serving.

Use caution when puréeing a hot soup. Cool slightly before puréeing, and avoid filling the blender or food processor more than three-quarters full.

6 servings

Prep Time:
30 minutes or less

Total Time:
30 minutes or less

Nutritional Information
Per Serving (about 1 cup)
Calories 125
Total Fat . . . . 3 g
Total Carbohydrate . . . . . . 20 g
Dietary Fiber . . . . 2 g
Sugars . . . . 6 g
Protein . . . . 5 g
Sodium . . . . 235 mg

Yukon Gold or Idaho potatoes are good options for this soup, but if you can't find those in your market, any kind of potato will work.

3 medium potatoes, peeled and cut into 1- to 2-inch pieces
2 celery stalks, cut into 1- to 2-inch pieces
½ onion, cut into 1-inch pieces
2 cups reduced-sodium chicken broth or vegetable broth
1 tablespoon butter
1 tablespoon all-purpose flour
2 cups low-fat milk
Salt and freshly ground black pepper

1. In a large saucepan over high heat, bring the potatoes, celery, onion, and broth to a boil. Reduce the heat, cover, and simmer for 15 to 20 minutes, or until the potatoes are tender, stirring occasionally. Cool slightly. Transfer to a blender or food processor and purée. Set aside.

2. In the same saucepan over low heat, melt the butter. Add the flour and cook until fully incorporated, stirring constantly. Gradually add the milk and cook until thickened, stirring constantly. Add the reserved potato mixture to the saucepan and stir well to combine. Season with salt and pepper.

Adapted, with permission, from *Eating Well, Staying Well During and After Cancer* (Atlanta, GA: American Cancer Society, 2004), 223.

Sherbet Shake

This refreshing shake is a cinch to make and offers lots of calories and protein too. If you're lactose intolerant, substitute lactose-free milk and sorbet for milk and sherbet in this recipe. Use orange sherbet for Creamsicle-like flavor.

1 serving

Prep Time:
15 minutes or less

Total Time:
15 minutes or less

Nutritional Information
Per Serving
Calories 320
Total Fat . . . . 4 g
Total Carbohydrate . . . . . . 63 g
Dietary Fiber . . . . 1 g
Sugars . . . . 61 g
Protein . . . . 8 g
Sodium . . . . 120 mg

1 cup sherbet
³/₄ cup low-fat milk
¹/₂ teaspoon vanilla extract

1. In a blender, combine the sherbet, milk, and vanilla and blend until smooth.

Adapted, with permission, from *Eating Well, Staying Well During and After Cancer* (Atlanta, GA: American Cancer Society, 2004), 211.

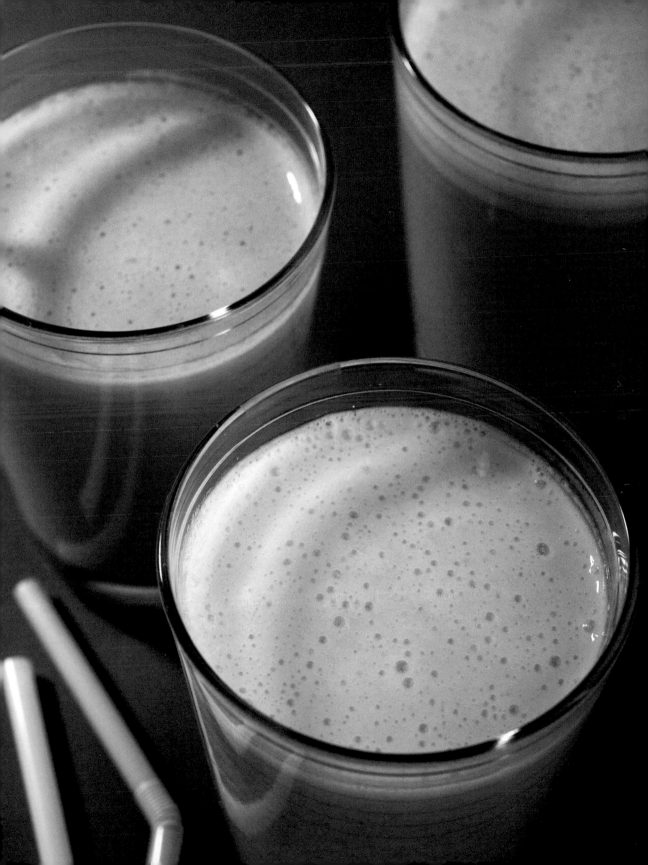

Creamy Frozen Fruit Bars

These easy-to-prepare dessert bars are made with just three ingredients. Let them soften slightly before serving so they are easier to cut. These are good when your mouth is bothering you or you need a cold, mildly flavored snack. Serve with fresh fruit as a dessert.

9 servings

Prep Time:
15 minutes or less

Total Time:
**15 minutes or less
plus 1 or more hours
freezing**

**Nutritional Information
Per Serving**
Calories 150
Total Fat . . . . 8 g
Total Carbohydrate . . . . . . 14 g
Dietary Fiber . . . . 0 g
Sugars . . . . 12 g
Protein . . . . 3 g
Sodium . . . . 115 mg

1 cup vanilla low-fat yogurt
½ cup all-fruit preserves
1 (8-ounce) package regular or reduced-fat cream cheese

1. Line an 8-by-8-inch pan with plastic wrap.

2. In a blender or food processor, combine the yogurt, preserves, and cream cheese and blend until smooth. Pour into the pan. Cover and freeze for 1 or more hours, or until firm.

3. Remove the mixture from the pan by lifting the plastic wrap. Let soften slightly, cut into squares, and serve. Refreeze what you aren't serving for later.

Adapted, with permission, from *Eating Well, Staying Well During and After Cancer* (Atlanta, GA: American Cancer Society, 2004), 236.

Tangy Protein Smoothie

This thick, protein-packed drink gets tanginess from cottage cheese. You can also substitute plain or flavored yogurt if you prefer.

When you are looking for an alternate protein source, cottage cheese is a good choice. One half cup has almost as much protein as 2 ounces of meat.

1 serving

Prep Time:
15 minutes or less

Total Time:
15 minutes or less

**Nutritional Information
Per Serving**
Calories 275
Total Fat . . . . 11 g
Total Carbohydrate . . . . . . 31 g
Dietary Fiber . . . . 1 g
Sugars . . . . 28 g
Protein . . . . 13 g
Sodium . . . . 380 mg

To make this in a jiffy, use individual snack packs of flavored gelatin.

Use leftover cottage cheese to make Creamy Mac and Cheese (page 121).

⅓ **cup cottage cheese or plain yogurt**
½ **cup vanilla ice cream**
¼ **cup prepared fruit-flavored gelatin**
¼ **cup low-fat milk**

1. In a blender, combine the cottage cheese, ice cream, gelatin, and milk and blend until smooth.

Adapted, with permission, from *Eating Well, Staying Well During and After Cancer* (Atlanta, GA: American Cancer Society, 2004), 211.

Carrot-Ginger Soup

Using a food processor to chop the vegetables makes the prep time super quick for this soup. Use quick pulses just until the onion is chopped to prevent it from getting mushy. Once you've started cooking the onion, chop the carrots. There's no need to worry about getting the sizes just right since the soup is puréed after cooking.

For a milder soup, reduce or eliminate the amount of ginger used.

Be very careful when puréeing a hot soup. Cool slightly before puréeing and avoid filling the blender or food processor more than three-quarters full.

5 servings

Prep Time:
15 minutes or less

Total Time:
1 hour or less

**Nutritional Information
Per Serving (about 1 cup)**
Calories 105
Total Fat . . . . 5 g
Total Carbohydrate . . . . . . 13 g
Dietary Fiber . . . . 3 g
Sugars . . . . 6 g
Protein . . . . 3 g
Sodium . . . . 490 mg

> Add calories by increasing the amount of cream used to 1 cup. If you are trying to lose weight, omit the cream.

2 garlic cloves

1 (1¼-inch) piece fresh ginger, peeled

1 onion, quartered

2 tablespoons butter or vegetable oil

1 pound carrots, cut into 1- to 2-inch pieces, or a 1-pound bag baby carrots, rinsed

4 cups reduced-sodium chicken broth

½ cup heavy cream, optional

Salt and freshly ground black pepper

1. In a food processor, with the motor running, drop in the garlic and ginger and purée. Stop the machine, add the onion, and pulse until evenly chopped.

2. In a stockpot over medium heat, melt the butter. Sauté the onion mixture for 5 to 8 minutes, or until softened.

3. Meanwhile, pulse the carrots in the food processor until finely chopped. Add to the onion mixture and sauté for 3 to 5 minutes. Add the broth and stir to combine. Bring to a boil. Reduce the heat, partially cover, and simmer for 30 to 40 minutes, or until very tender, stirring occasionally. Stir in the cream. Cool slightly.

4. Transfer to a blender or food processor and purée (you may need to do this step in two or more batches). Season with salt and pepper.

Hearty Turkey Minestrone Soup

This soup is chock-full of veggies, pasta, beans, and meat. You might need to add more broth when reheating leftovers—the pasta will absorb the liquid.

14 servings

Prep Time:
30 minutes or less

Total Time:
1 hour or less

Nutritional Information
Per Serving (about 1 cup)
Calories 120
Total Fat . . . . 1 g
Total Carbohydrate . . . . . . 15 g
Dietary Fiber . . . . 3 g
Sugars . . . . 4 g
Protein . . . . 13 g
Sodium . . . . 420 mg

1 pound ground turkey breast or lean ground beef
1 onion, chopped
2 carrots, chopped
2 celery stalks, chopped
8 cups reduced-sodium chicken broth or beef broth
1 (14.5-ounce) can diced tomatoes
1 teaspoon dried basil
1 teaspoon dried oregano
½ cup small pasta, such as orzo or pastini
1 (10-ounce) package frozen chopped spinach
1 (15-ounce) can chickpeas or white beans, rinsed and drained
Salt and freshly ground black pepper
Grated Parmesan cheese, optional

1. In a stockpot over medium-high heat, sauté the turkey and onion until the turkey is cooked through. Add the carrots and celery and sauté for 10 minutes, or until softened. Add the broth, tomatoes, basil, and oregano and stir to combine. Bring to a boil. Reduce the heat and simmer for 20 minutes, stirring occasionally.

2. Add the pasta, frozen spinach, and chickpeas and cook for 10 minutes, or until pasta is tender, stirring occasionally. Season with salt and pepper. Serve with Parmesan cheese.

Adapted, with permission, from *Eating Well, Staying Well During and After Cancer* (Atlanta, GA: American Cancer Society, 2004), 219.

Roasted Root Vegetable Soup

Using roasted vegetables takes much of the effort out of making homemade soup. Just spread the veggies on baking sheets and let the oven's heat transform them into creamy, soft, caramelized gems. Purée them with broth and the soup's on! Precise measurements aren't necessary; just add enough broth to make the soup as thick or thin as you like.

Depending on the size of your food processor, you might need to purée the vegetables in batches. If so, transfer the puréed mixture to a large bowl before adding all the broth.

Most supermarkets now sell small butternut squash, which are the perfect size for making this soup.

7 servings

Prep Time:
15 minutes or less

Total Time:
1 hour or less

Nutritional Information
Per Serving (about 1 cup)
Calories 100
Total Fat . . . . 4 g
Total Carbohydrate . . . . . . 14 g
Dietary Fiber . . . . 2 g
Sugars . . . . 6 g
Protein . . . . 3 g
Sodium . . . . 320 mg

3 carrots, cut into 1-inch pieces
1 small (about 1 pound) butternut squash, peeled and seeded, cut into 1¼-inch pieces
1 small (about 8 ounces) sweet potato, peeled and cut into 1¼-inch pieces
1 small sweet onion, peeled and cut into 1¼-inch pieces
2 tablespoons olive oil
Salt and freshly ground black pepper
5 cups reduced-sodium chicken broth or vegetable broth, heated

1. Preheat the oven to 400 degrees.

2. On two foil-lined, rimmed baking sheets, combine the carrots, squash, sweet potato, and onion. Drizzle with oil and toss to coat. Sprinkle with salt and pepper. Roast for 40 to 50 minutes, or until very tender and slightly charred, tossing every 15 minutes.

3. Transfer to a food processor and add 3 cups of the warmed broth. Blend until smooth, adding more of the broth to achieve desired consistency. (You may need to do this step in batches or transfer the mixture to a large bowl before adding all the broth.)

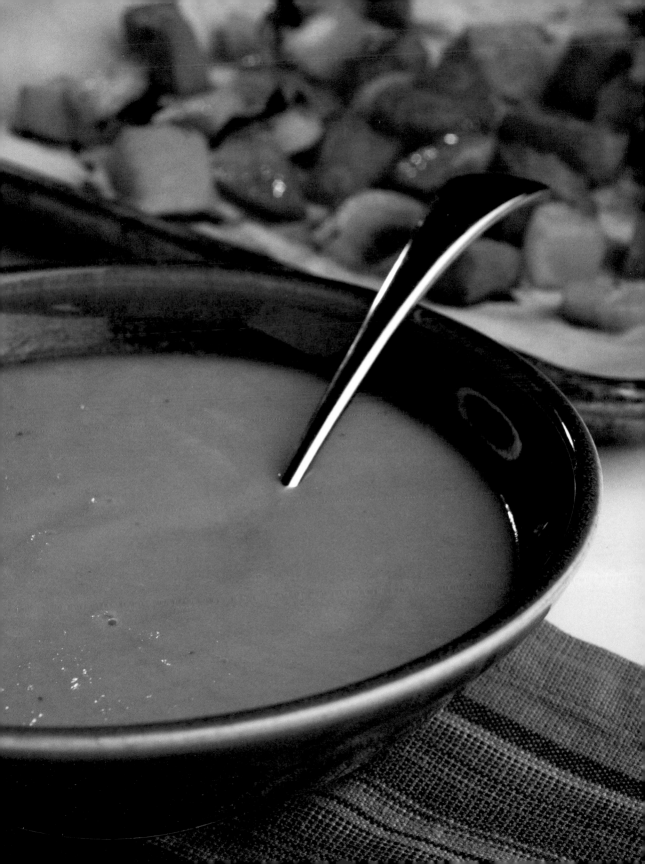

Fruity Drink

Making your own juice with a juicer ensures you'll get nutrients and liquids while avoiding the preservatives and refined sugars that are in many store-bought juices.

Keep frozen berries on hand for making this drink.

3 servings

Prep Time:
15 minutes or less

Total Time:
15 minutes or less

Nutritional Information
Per Serving (about 1 small cup)
Calories 110
Total Fat . . . . 1 g
Total Carbohydrate . . . . . . 28 g
Dietary Fiber . . . . 1 g
Sugars . . . . 19 g
Protein . . . . 2 g
Sodium . . . . 0 mg

This recipe may not be
appropriate if you have
mouth sores.

12 green or red grapes
6 large strawberries, hulled
3 slices pineapple
1 apple
½ ripe banana, peeled
½ orange or tangerine, peeled
½ cup fresh or frozen raspberries
½ cup fresh or frozen blackberries

1. In a juicer, combine the grapes, strawberries, pineapple, apple, banana, orange, raspberries, and blackberries, and process according to machine directions.

Adapted, with permission, from *Eating Well, Staying Well During and After Cancer* (Atlanta, GA: American Cancer Society, 2004), 210.

Veggie Drink

This vegetable juice will help you replenish necessary nutrients and liquids. Make sure you wash all the vegetables really well. There's no need for other prep.

Red or yellow peppers enhance the sweetness of the drink.

2 servings

Prep Time:
15 minutes or less

Total Time:
15 minutes or less

Nutritional Information
Per Serving (about 1 small cup)
Calories 110
Total Fat . . . . 1 g
Total Carbohydrate . . . . . . 25 g
Dietary Fiber . . . . 3 g
Sugars . . . . 13 g
Protein . . . . 4 g
Sodium . . . . 180 mg

4 carrots
3 broccoli florets with stems
2 celery stalks
1 beet, halved
½ green bell pepper
¼ head of cabbage
Handful of spinach
Handful of Italian parsley

1. In a juicer, combine the carrots, broccoli, celery, beet, green pepper, cabbage, spinach, and parsley, and process according to machine directions.

Adapted, with permission, from *Eating Well, Staying Well During and After Cancer* (Atlanta, GA: American Cancer Society, 2004), 210.

TASTE ALTERATIONS

Chemotherapy, radiation therapy, and certain medications may change the way you taste and smell foods. It can be difficult to get the calories and nutrients you need when foods no longer taste and smell the way you remember them. Alterations in taste and smell typically resolve themselves a few months after treatment ends.

You may find that food has a metallic or bitter taste or no taste at all. Food may taste too salty or sweet. Your old favorites may not be appealing, and now may be a good time to try new and different flavors.

• Foods such as meat, coffee, and chocolate may taste different from usual.

• If meat does not taste good, look for alternative sources of protein, such as eggs, dairy, beans or peas, nuts and nut butters, seeds and high-protein bread and pasta.

• To lessen problems with metallic tastes, use plastic utensils instead of metal, choose fresh or frozen foods instead of canned foods, and microwave or bake in glass or ceramic cookware.

• Add lemon juice or vinegar to vegetables to mask metallic or bitter tastes.

• Marinate meats in Italian salad dressing, mustard, or barbecue, soy, or teriyaki sauce.

• Sour foods such as cranberries, cranberry juice, sauerkraut, pickles, and pickled beets or okra may offer more flavor.

• Foods with strong flavors, such as onions, garlic, and feta or Parmesan cheese, may be able to cut through the "blah" taste. Feel free to increase the amounts of spices in recipes if it suits your tastes.

• Sugar-free candies like mints or lemon drops may mask unpleasant tastes.

(N)	Nausea
(D)	Diarrhea
(C)	Constipation
(SM)	Sore Mouth and Difficulty Swallowing
(TA)	Taste Alterations
(WL)	Unintentional Weight Loss

• Fresh and frozen vegetables may be more appealing than canned ones.

• Fruit smoothies and frozen desserts like sorbet or sherbet may be appealing.

Experiment with different flavors and temperatures to see what works best for you.

Consider rinsing your mouth with a mixture of 4 cups water, 1 teaspoon baking soda, and ¾ teaspoon salt throughout the day to reduce unpleasant tastes.

For more information about managing changes in taste, contact the American Cancer Society at 800-227-2345 or visit our Web site at cancer.org.

Chai Latte

This milky tea drink is flavored with aromatic spices that are calming to the stomach. It's a coffeehouse favorite that is easy to prepare at home.

A small seedpod, cardamom is a spice that is often used in baking and in Indian cuisine. It is available in spice markets, specialty stores, and mail-order outlets.

2 servings

Prep Time:
15 minutes or less

Total Time:
15 minutes or less

**Nutritional Information
Per Serving (about ¾ cup)**
Calories 90
Total Fat . . . . 1 g
Total Carbohydrate . . . . . . 17 g
Dietary Fiber . . . . 0 g
Sugars . . . . 16 g
Protein . . . . 3 g
Sodium . . . . 40 mg

Low-fat milk has less saturated fat than whole milk, without the thin consistency of nonfat milk.

²/₃ **cup low-fat milk**
6 cardamom pods
5 whole cloves
4 black peppercorns
1 (about 1½ inches long) cinnamon stick
¼ teaspoon vanilla extract
1 tea bag
1 cup boiling water
2 to 3 tablespoons granulated sugar

1. In a saucepan over low heat, combine the milk, cardamom, cloves, peppercorns, cinnamon stick, and vanilla. Simmer for 5 minutes.

2. Meanwhile, in a mug, combine the tea bag and boiling water. Let steep for 5 minutes.

3. Remove the milk from the heat and stir in 2 tablespoons of the sugar until dissolved. Remove the tea bag and fill mug with strained hot milk mixture. Taste and add the remaining tablespoon sugar if needed.

Smoked Salmon Spread

This full-flavored dip will tickle your taste buds with its interplay of smoky fish, briny capers, and vibrant fresh herbs. For a light meal, smear the spread on crackers or bagel crisps, or for a more substantial meal, use it as a sandwich filling. For added zing, add a dash of horseradish.

8 servings

Prep Time:
15 minutes or less

Total Time:
15 minutes or less

Nutritional Information
Per Serving
(about 2 tablespoons)
Calories 60
Total Fat . . . . 5 g
Total Carbohydrate . . . . 1 g
Dietary Fiber . . . . 0 g
Sugars . . . . 1 g
Protein . . . . 4 g
Sodium . . . . 200 mg

If you have mouth sores, omit the lemon juice and capers.

This recipe may not be appropriate for immuno-compromised patients.

½ **(8-ounce) tub regular or reduced-fat cream cheese**
4 ounces smoked salmon, chopped, divided
1 tablespoon fresh lemon juice
2 tablespoons chopped fresh dill
1 heaping tablespoon chopped capers
1 heaping tablespoon finely chopped red onion or chives

1. In a food processor, pulse the cream cheese, half of the smoked salmon, and lemon juice until smooth.

2. Transfer to a bowl and stir in the remaining salmon, dill, capers, and red onion.

Gazpacho

This chilled soup is filled with healthy vegetables and provides nutrients and bright flavor in a bowl. To speed prep time, use a food processor for chopping your vegetables and mixing. You may need to do this step in two or more batches, depending on the size of your food processor. To chop the vegetables (without pulverizing them) use the pulse button.

The vegetables can also be chopped by hand.

10 servings

Prep Time:
30 minutes or less

Total Time:
30 minutes or less
plus 2 or more hours
refrigeration

Nutritional Information
Per Serving (about 1 cup)
Calories 65
Total Fat . . . . 3 g
Total Carbohydrate . . . . . . 10 g
Dietary Fiber . . . . 2 g
Sugars . . . . 6 g
Protein . . . . 2 g
Sodium . . . . 870 mg

Canned tomatoes are better than fresh ones as a source of the antioxidant lycopene.

This recipe may not be appropriate for those who are experiencing gas.

1 large garlic clove
1 small (or ½ large) red onion, cut into 1- to 2-inch pieces
1 green bell pepper, seeded and cut into 1- to 2-inch pieces
1 red bell pepper, seeded and cut into 1- to 2-inch pieces
1 cucumber, peeled, seeded, and cut into 1- to 2-inch pieces
1 (28-ounce) can Italian plum tomatoes
2 tablespoons olive oil
2 tablespoons red wine vinegar
2 teaspoons salt
1 teaspoon granulated sugar
½ teaspoon ground black pepper
Tabasco or other hot red pepper sauce
2 cups tomato juice or tomato-vegetable juice

1. In a food processor, with the motor running, drop in the garlic and purée. Stop the machine, add the onion, and pulse until coarsely chopped. Add both bell peppers and cucumber and pulse until coarsely chopped. Add the tomatoes, oil, vinegar, salt, sugar, black pepper, and a few shakes of Tabasco and pulse until all of the vegetables are chopped but still chunky, about 30 seconds. Do not overprocess.

2. Transfer to a large bowl. Add the tomato juice and stir to combine. Cover and refrigerate for at least 2 hours before serving.

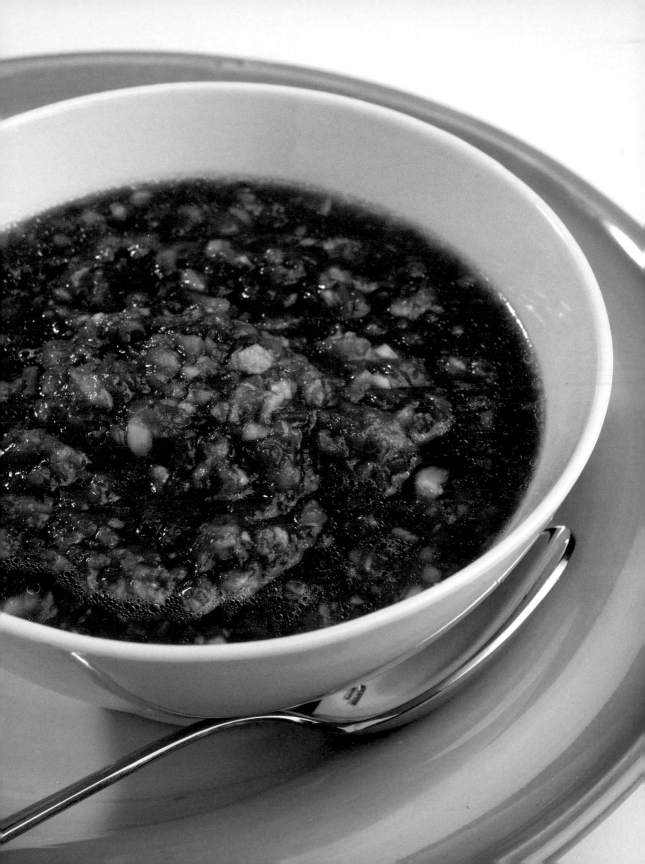

Microwaved Lemon-Spiked Chicken with Mushrooms

This microwaved dish comes together very quickly. Even better, the only effort required is stirring it every few minutes.

The light lemon flavor compliments the combination of chicken and mushrooms. If you're looking for more assertive flavor, season with tarragon, an herb with a licorice-like flavor. Serve over rice or pasta.

6 servings

Prep Time:
15 minutes or less

Total Time:
30 minutes or less

Nutritional Information
Per Serving
Calories 180
Total Fat . . . . 7 g
Total Carbohydrate . . . . 2 g
Dietary Fiber . . . . 0 g
Sugars . . . . 1 g
Protein . . . . 26 g
Sodium . . . . 110 mg

8 ounces mushrooms, sliced

1 teaspoon plus 2 tablespoons butter, divided

1½ pounds boneless, skinless chicken breasts, cut into 2-inch pieces

1 tablespoon all-purpose flour

½ teaspoon dried tarragon, optional

Salt and freshly ground black pepper

¼ cup reduced-sodium chicken broth

½ lemon, thinly sliced

1. In a microwave-safe bowl, combine the mushrooms and 1 teaspoon of the butter. Cover with plastic wrap and microwave on high for 1½ minutes, stirring after 1 minute.

2. Place the remaining 2 tablespoons butter in an 8-by-8-inch or 8-by-11-inch microwave-safe casserole dish and microwave on high for 45 to 60 seconds, or until melted. Add the chicken in a single layer and sprinkle with flour, tarragon, salt, and pepper.

3. Cover with plastic wrap and microwave on high for 4 minutes, stirring at 1-minute intervals. Add the mushrooms and broth and arrange lemon slices on top. Microwave on high for 5 minutes, or until chicken is tender. Season with salt and pepper.

Adapted, with permission, from *The American Cancer Society's Healthy Eating Cookbook, Third Edition* (Atlanta, GA: American Cancer Society, 2005), 72.

Crunchy Asian Salad

This salad features the crunch of uncooked ramen noodles and shredded cabbage. For a more colorful presentation, choose a coleslaw blend of red and green cabbage and shredded carrots.

For variety, add pineapple chunks, sliced almonds, or sesame seeds.

Crushing the ramen into small pieces while it's still in the package keeps the mess to a minimum. Reserve the seasoning packet to add to the dressing. The packet contains a lot of sodium, so add a little at a time until it suits your taste.

9 servings

Prep Time:
15 minutes or less

Total Time:
15 minutes or less

Nutritional Information
Per Serving (about ½ cup)
Calories 155
Total Fat . . . . 11 g
Total Carbohydrate . . . . . . 14 g
Dietary Fiber . . . . 1 g
Sugars . . . . 7 g
Protein . . . . 1 g
Sodium . . . . 210 mg

Olive oil is rich in monounsaturated fat, a heart healthy fat.

1 (3-ounce) package ramen noodles (chicken or other flavor), crushed, seasoning packet reserved
3 cups (about half of a 10-ounce package) coleslaw mix
3 scallions, thinly sliced
1 (11-ounce) can mandarin oranges, drained
6 tablespoons olive oil
3 tablespoons balsamic vinegar
3 tablespoons granulated sugar

1. In a bowl, combine the ramen noodles, coleslaw mix, scallions, and oranges.

2. In a separate bowl, combine the oil, vinegar, sugar, and ramen seasoning packet to taste. Add to the salad and stir gently to incorporate.

Adapted, with permission, from *Eating Well, Staying Well During and After Cancer* (Atlanta, GA: American Cancer Society, 2004), 224.

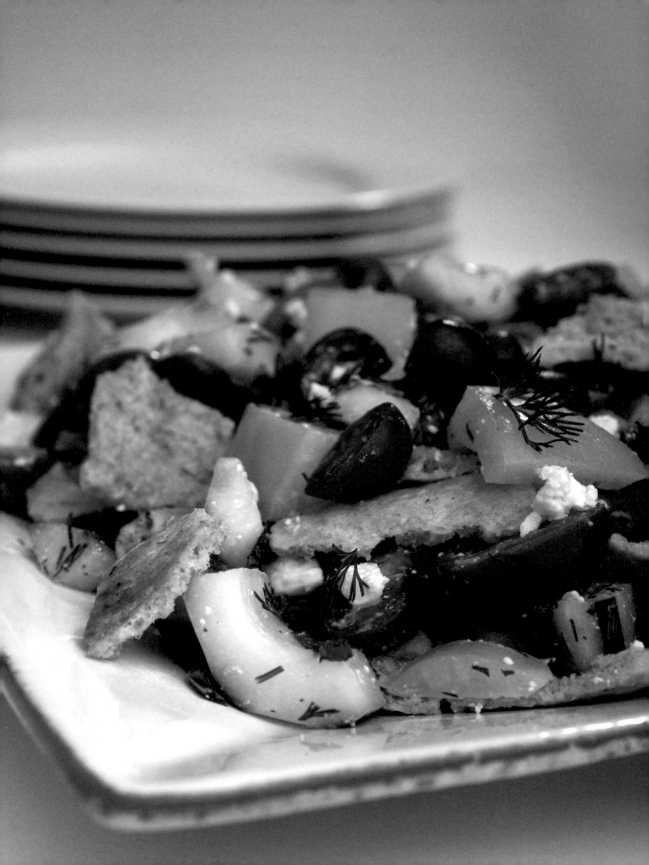

Veggie–Pita Bread Salad

This chunky salad is loaded with colorful veggies and herbs. The addition of toasted bread and feta cheese gives it extra heft and protein. As the salad sits, the flavors meld and the bread softens.

The recipe can also be halved.

7 servings

Prep Time:
30 minutes or less

Total Time:
30 minutes or less

Nutritional Information
Per Serving (about 1 cup)
Calories 145
Total Fat . . . . 10 g
Total Carbohydrate . . . . . . 11 g
Dietary Fiber . . . . 2 g
Sugars . . . . 3 g
Protein . . . . 5 g
Sodium . . . . 360 mg

1 pint grape tomatoes, halved

1 cucumber, peeled, seeded, and cut into bite-sized pieces

1 red, yellow, or green bell pepper, seeded and cut into bite-sized pieces

2 tablespoons finely chopped red onion

15 kalamata olives, pitted and chopped

1 whole wheat or plain pita bread, toasted, split, and cut into bite-sized pieces

1 cup crumbled feta cheese

¼ cup chopped fresh mint

2 tablespoons chopped fresh dill

2 to 3 tablespoons olive oil

1 to 2 tablespoons red wine vinegar

Salt and freshly ground black pepper

1. In a bowl, combine the tomatoes, cucumber, bell pepper, and onion. Add the olives, pita bread, feta cheese, mint, and dill.

2. In a separate bowl, combine 2 tablespoons of the oil and 1 tablespoon of the red wine vinegar. Add to the salad and stir gently to incorporate. Season with salt and pepper. Add more oil or vinegar if necessary.

Tuna-Bean Salad

This non-mayonnaise–based salad pairs the protein-packed combo of tuna and beans with lots of fresh crunchy veggies.

For stronger flavor, add another can of tuna or mix in sliced kalamata olives or feta cheese. For more protein, add in a chopped hard-boiled egg or two.

6 servings

Prep Time:
15 minutes or less

Total Time:
15 minutes or less

**Nutritional Information
Per Serving (about ½ cup)**
Calories 180
Total Fat . . . . 6 g
Total Carbohydrate . . . . . . 17 g
Dietary Fiber . . . . 5 g
Sugars . . . . 5 g
Protein . . . . 14 g
Sodium . . . . 400 mg

> If you're watching calories, choose a "light" dressing.
>
> For fresher flavor, make your own dressing. Mix ¼ cup balsamic vinegar or fresh lemon juice and 3 to 4 tablespoons extra-virgin olive oil.

2 (5-ounce) cans white tuna packed in water, drained
2 scallions, thinly sliced
1 tomato, chopped
1 red bell pepper, seeded and chopped
1 carrot, chopped
1 celery stalk, chopped
1 (15-ounce) can chickpeas, rinsed and drained
¼ cup chopped fresh Italian parsley, optional
⅓ cup balsamic vinaigrette or other dressing
Salt and freshly ground black pepper

1. In a bowl, flake the tuna. Add the scallions, tomato, red pepper, carrot, celery, chickpeas, and parsley and stir to combine. Drizzle with vinaigrette and stir gently to incorporate. Season with salt and pepper.

Chicken Picatta

This elegant entrée gets tartness from lemons and a little zing from briny capers. Buying packaged "thin-sliced" boneless chicken breasts ensures uniform cooking time and provides just the right portion size.

For more acidity, add lemon juice, zest, or sliced lemons. For an herbal note, top with chopped fresh Italian parsley.

Avoid using a nonstick skillet when making dishes that include a pan gravy, such as this one. When you deglaze the skillet by adding liquid, you'll incorporate flavor from the caramelized cooked chicken that has adhered to the pan.

4 servings

Prep Time:
15 minutes or less

Total Time:
30 minutes or less

Nutritional Information
Per Serving
Calories 225
Total Fat . . . . 10 g
Total Carbohydrate . . . . 8 g
Dietary Fiber . . . . 0 g
Sugars . . . . 1 g
Protein . . . . 26 g
Sodium . . . . 310 mg

To increase calories, add a few tablespoons of heavy cream to the sauce before returning the chicken to the pan.

¼ cup all-purpose flour
Salt and freshly ground black pepper
1 pound "thin-sliced" boneless, skinless chicken breasts or full-sized breasts pounded to even thickness
2 tablespoons olive oil
2 garlic cloves, finely chopped
1 cup reduced-sodium chicken broth
Juice of 1 lemon
2 tablespoons capers

1. On a plate, combine the flour and a sprinkle of salt and pepper. Lightly dredge the chicken in the flour.

2. In a large skillet over medium-high heat, add the oil. Sauté the garlic for 1 minute. Add the chicken and cook for 3 to 5 minutes per side, or until golden and just cooked through. Remove the chicken and set aside.

3. Add the broth and lemon juice to the skillet and bring to a boil. Boil until the sauce has reduced by about half, scraping up any browned bits clinging to the pan.

4. Return the chicken to the skillet, add the capers, and cook for 2 to 3 minutes, or until heated through. Season with salt and pepper.

Pita Pesto Pizzas

Store-bought pesto, a combination of basil, garlic, olive oil, and Parmesan cheese, offers an effortless burst of flavor. While primarily eaten as a pasta topping, it can also be used as a condiment. It can usually be found in the refrigerated section or the pasta aisle of most supermarkets. If possible, get the refrigerated variety—it has a fresher, more authentic flavor.

Feta cheese and olives add zip without being overpowering.

This flavorful dish can be eaten as a meal, snack, or appetizer.

2 servings

Prep Time:
15 minutes or less

Total Time:
30 minutes or less

Nutritional Information
Per Serving
Calories 225
Total Fat . . . . 11 g
Total Carbohydrate . . . . . . 22 g
Dietary Fiber . . . . 4 g
Sugars . . . . 3 g
Protein . . . . 11 g
Sodium . . . . 650 mg

1 whole wheat or plain pita, split open
2 tablespoons prepared pesto
6 to 8 slices ripe tomato
¼ cup crumbled feta cheese
¼ cup shredded mozzarella cheese
2 tablespoons sliced black olives, optional

1. Preheat the oven to 400 degrees. Line a rimmed baking sheet with foil.

2. Place pitas, rough side up, on the baking sheet and spread each half with 1 tablespoon pesto. Top each piece with tomato slices. Sprinkle with feta and mozzarella cheeses and olives.

3. Bake for 10 minutes, or until cheese melts and bread crisps.

Turkey Roll-Up with Cranberry-Orange Relish

A citrus-cranberry relish adds piquancy to an easy roll-up sandwich. Make your own or look for a prepared jar at the market. Slice and have it ready in the fridge for when you feel up to eating.

If your mouth can handle crunchy vegetables, top the turkey with shredded carrots and chopped lettuce before rolling. Omit the relish if your mouth is sensitive.

1 serving

Prep Time:
15 minutes or less

Total Time:
15 minutes or less

**Nutritional Information
Per Serving**
Calories 300
Total Fat . . . . 4.5 g
Total Carbohydrate . . . . . . 46 g
Dietary Fiber . . . . 4 g
Sugars . . . . 18 g
Protein . . . . 18 g
Sodium . . . . 530 mg

Use leftover relish to top Mini Turkey Burgers (page 129).

½ unpeeled orange, seeded and halved

½ unpeeled apple, seeded and halved

1 (16-ounce) can whole cranberry sauce

1 (8-inch) whole wheat or plain flour tortilla or flatbread such as lavash

2 large slices (about 1½ ounces) roasted turkey breast or rotisserie chicken breast

1. In a food processor, pulse the orange until coarsely chopped. Add the apple and pulse until both are finely chopped. Transfer to a bowl and add cranberry sauce, stirring well to combine.

2. Spread ¼ cup of the cranberry mixture over tortilla. Layer the turkey on half of the tortilla. Roll up jellyroll style, beginning with the meat side. Slice into 2-inch pieces.

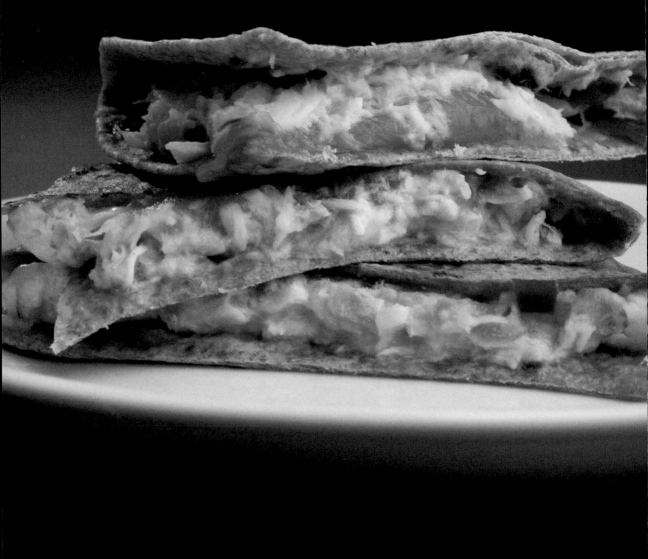

Tuna Melt Quesadilla

This twist on a classic gives new life to the tuna melt. A quesadilla is a good choice when a sandwich seems overwhelming.

Choose full-fat options if trying to gain weight, reduced-fat if you are watching calories.

3 servings

Prep Time:
15 minutes or less

Total Time:
15 minutes or less

Nutritional Information
Per Serving (1 quesadilla)
Calories 360
Total Fat . . . . 17 g
Total Carbohydrate . . . . . . 31 g
Dietary Fiber . . . . 3 g
Sugars . . . . 3 g
Protein . . . . 21 g
Sodium . . . . 940 mg

Microwaving the quesadilla instead of pan-frying or baking keeps it softer.

1 (5-ounce) can tuna in water, drained
1 tablespoon regular or reduced-fat mayonnaise
½ tablespoon Dijon mustard
1 tablespoon finely chopped red onion
1 tablespoon pickle relish
3 (8-inch) whole wheat or plain tortillas
¾ cup shredded regular or reduced-fat Cheddar or "Mexican-style" cheese

1. In a bowl, flake the tuna. Add the mayonnaise and mustard and stir to combine. Add the onion and relish.

2. On a microwave-safe plate, place 1 tortilla and spread half with ⅓ of the tuna mixture. Sprinkle the other half with ¼ cup cheese. Fold the tuna half over the cheese half. Microwave on high for 40 to 50 seconds, or until cheese melts. Repeat twice with the remaining ingredients.

Orange Beef, Asparagus, and Mushroom Stir-Fry

A stir-fry offers the cook flexibility to customize a dish to suit individual preferences. You can substitute chicken, tofu, or pork for the beef. Add bell peppers or other vegetables to increase fiber.

Oyster sauce, available in the international food aisle of most supermarkets, adds a lot of flavor and can stand up to assertive vegetables such as asparagus.

4 servings

Prep Time:
15 minutes or less

Total Time:
30 minutes or less

Nutritional Information
Per Serving
Calories 225
Total Fat . . . . 8 g
Total Carbohydrate . . . . . . 12 g
Dietary Fiber . . . . 3 g
Sugars . . . . 1 g
Protein . . . . 26 g
Sodium . . . . 880 mg

1 tablespoon vegetable oil

3 garlic cloves, finely chopped

¼ teaspoon crushed red pepper flakes, or to taste

1 pound asparagus, trimmed and sliced diagonally into bite-sized pieces

1 pound sirloin steak or other lean beef, trimmed of excess fat and thinly sliced

2 (4-ounce) packages sliced wild mushrooms or 8 ounces shiitake or other mushrooms, stemmed and sliced

½ cup oyster sauce

Zest of 1 orange

1. In a wok or large skillet over high heat, add the oil. Sauté the garlic and red pepper flakes for 1 minute. Add the asparagus and sauté for 3 to 5 minutes. Add the beef and mushrooms and sauté for 3 to 5 minutes. If mixture is drying out, add 1 to 2 tablespoons water. Add the oyster sauce and orange zest and stir to combine. Sauté for 1 to 2 minutes, or until the vegetables and beef are cooked through.

Sweet and Sour Meatballs

A little more sweet than sour, these meatballs simmer in a rich and succulent tomato-based sauce. Serve over rice or egg noodles moistened with the sauce.

To make the meatballs more "sour," increase the amount of vinegar.

4 servings

Prep Time:
30 minutes or less

Total Time:
1 hour and 30 minutes or less

Nutritional Information
Per Serving
(about 5 meatballs)
Calories 435
Total Fat . . . . 15 g
Total Carbohydrate . . . . . . 52 g
Dietary Fiber . . . . 3 g
Sugars . . . . 44 g
Protein . . . . 25 g
Sodium . . . . 960 mg

1 slice white bread, crust removed

⅓ cup low-fat milk

1 pound lean ground beef (preferably 93 percent lean) or ground turkey breast

½ teaspoon salt

½ teaspoon ground black pepper

2 tablespoons vegetable oil

1 small (or ½ large) onion, chopped

1 (15-ounce) can tomato sauce

½ cup (packed) light brown sugar

½ cup raisins

¼ cup white vinegar

1. In a bowl, soak the bread in milk until saturated. Squeeze the milk from the bread and discard the excess milk. Gently combine the bread, beef, salt, and pepper. Form the mixture into 1½-inch balls.

2. In a large skillet over medium heat, add the oil. Lightly brown the meatballs on all sides for 5 to 8 minutes (you may need to do this step in two or more batches).

3. Meanwhile, in a stockpot or deep skillet over medium heat, combine the onion, tomato sauce, brown sugar, raisins, and vinegar and bring to a simmer. When the meatballs are browned, add to the sauce and stir to combine. Cover and simmer for 30 minutes.

4. Uncover and simmer for an additional 20 to 30 minutes, or until the meat is cooked through and the sauce thickens, stirring occasionally.

Orzo Salad with Spinach, Tomatoes, and Feta

Orzo, rice-shaped pasta, makes a great base for this colorful red, white, and green pasta salad. If you don't have orzo on hand, the dish can also be made with other small, shaped pasta.

For a version that's lower in fat and calories, decrease the amount of cheese, oil, and nuts.

This recipe makes enough for a crowd, but can easily be halved or even quartered. If not eating all at once, reserve some nuts to sprinkle over the salad just before eating.

12 servings

Prep Time:
30 minutes or less

Total Time:
30 minutes or less

Nutritional Information
Per Serving (about 1 cup)
Calories 350
Total Fat . . . . 21 g
Total Carbohydrate . . . . . . 32 g
Dietary Fiber . . . . 3 g
Sugars . . . . 7 g
Protein . . . . 10 g
Sodium . . . . 300 mg

Lightly toasting the pine nuts gives them added flavor and crunch. Bake at 350 degrees for a few minutes or cook in a dry skillet until golden and aromatic. Watch to make sure they don't burn.

1 (16-ounce) package orzo or other shaped pasta
1 (10-ounce) bag baby spinach, washed and coarsely chopped
1 pint grape or cherry tomatoes, halved
2 cups (½ pound) crumbled feta cheese
½ red onion, chopped
½ cup chopped fresh basil, or to taste
½ cup olive oil
½ cup balsamic vinegar
Salt and freshly ground black pepper
¾ cup pine nuts, toasted

1. Prepare the orzo according to package directions. During the last minute of cooking, add the spinach to the pot. Drain and rinse with cold water.

2. Meanwhile, in a large bowl, combine the tomatoes, feta, onion, and basil. In a separate bowl, combine the oil and vinegar. Add the drained orzo mixture and the oil mixture to the tomatoes and stir gently to incorporate. Season with salt and pepper. Just before serving, top with pine nuts.

Adapted, with permission, from *Eating Well, Staying Well During and After Cancer* (Atlanta, GA: American Cancer Society, 2004), 224.

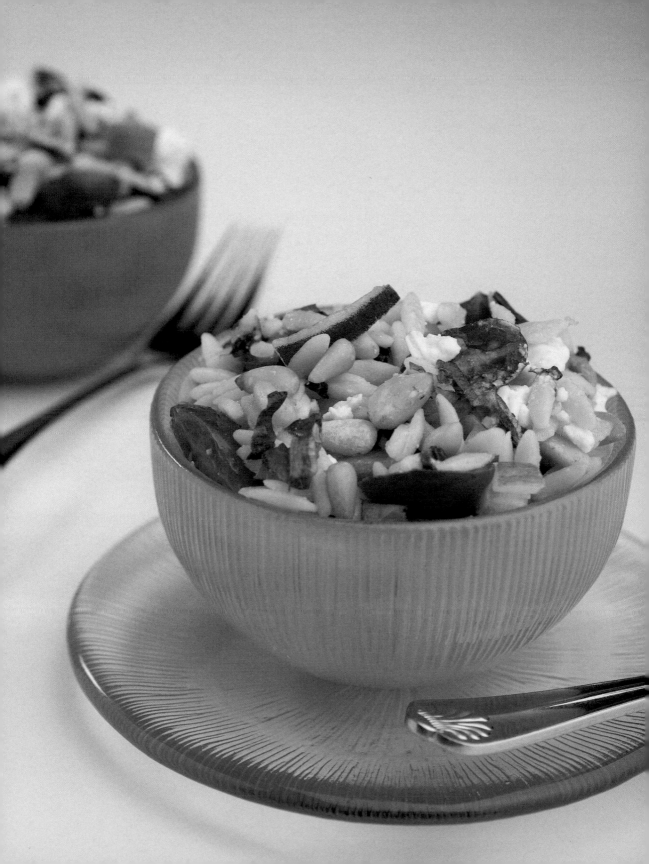

Citrus Tilapia

This light fish entrée gets a flavor boost from a citrus glaze made from fresh lemon juice, orange juice, and fresh ginger. For stronger, more acidic flavor, add lemon zest and additional juice. Make sure to use a high-quality 100 percent orange juice that is freshly squeezed (not from concentrate).

4 servings

Prep Time:
15 minutes or less

Total Time:
30 minutes or less

**Nutritional Information
Per Serving**

Calories 200
Total Fat . . . . 9 g
Total Carbohydrate . . . . 7 g
Dietary Fiber . . . . 0 g
Sugars . . . . 3 g
Protein . . . . 23 g
Sodium . . . . 55 mg

This recipe is not appropriate if you have mouth sores.

2 tablespoons all-purpose flour
Salt and freshly ground black pepper
1 pound tilapia fillets
1 tablespoon olive oil
1 tablespoon butter
½ cup freshly squeezed orange juice or high-quality store-bought orange juice
1 lemon, zested and juiced
½ teaspoon grated fresh ginger

1. On a plate, combine the flour and a sprinkle of salt and pepper. Lightly dredge the tilapia in the flour.

2. In a large skillet over medium heat, add the oil and butter. When the butter has melted, add the fish and cook for 2 to 3 minutes per side, or until golden and just cooked through. Remove the fish and set aside.

3. Add the orange juice, 2 tablespoons of the lemon juice, and the ginger to the skillet. Increase the heat and simmer for 1 to 2 minutes, or until thickened, stirring occasionally. Taste and add lemon zest or more lemon juice if necessary. Return the fish to the skillet, coat with sauce, and cook for 1 to 2 minutes, or until heated through.

Greek Chicken with Tomatoes, Peppers, Olives, and Feta

To add a lot of flavor with just one ingredient, look in the spice section for Greek seasoning, a mixture of dried onion, spearmint, oregano, and garlic. It adds lots of "oomph" to this quick and colorful dish.

During the warmer months, substitute ripe Roma tomatoes for canned.

4 servings

Prep Time:
30 minutes or less

Total Time:
30 minutes or less

**Nutritional Information
Per Serving**
Calories 265
Total Fat . . . . 9 g
Total Carbohydrate . . . . . . 17 g
Dietary Fiber . . . . 3 g
Sugars . . . . 6 g
Protein . . . . 28 g
Sodium . . . . 390 mg

¼ **cup all-purpose flour**
2 **tablespoons salt-free Greek seasoning, divided**
1 **pound boneless, skinless chicken breasts, cut into bite-sized pieces**
1 **to 2 tablespoons olive oil**
1 **onion, sliced lengthwise into strips**
1 **green bell pepper, seeded and sliced lengthwise into strips**
1 **(14.5-ounce) can diced tomatoes, partially drained, or 3 Roma tomatoes, cut into eighths**
¼ **cup pitted and chopped kalamata olives**
¼ **cup crumbled feta cheese**

1. On a plate, combine the flour and 1 tablespoon of the Greek seasoning. Lightly dredge the chicken in the flour.

2. In a large skillet over medium-high heat, add 1 tablespoon of the oil. Add the chicken and cook for 3 to 5 minutes per side, or until golden and just cooked through. Remove the chicken and set aside.

3. Add the onion to the skillet and sauté for 3 to 5 minutes, or until softened, adding more oil if necessary. Add the green pepper and sauté for 2 minutes. Add the tomatoes and the remaining 1 tablespoon Greek seasoning and cook for 5 minutes, stirring well to combine. Return the chicken to the skillet and cook for 1 to 2 minutes, or until heated through. Before serving, sprinkle with olives and feta.

Adapted, with permission, from *Celebrate! Healthy Entertaining for Any Occasion* (Atlanta, GA: American Cancer Society, 2001), 118.

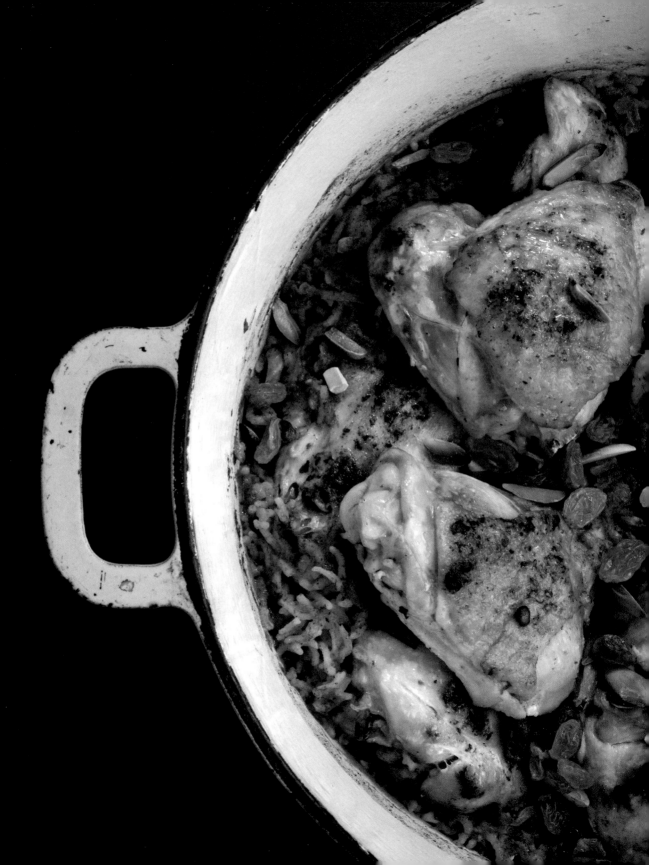

Curried Chicken and Rice

This fragrant curry dish provides a lot of flavor without being overpowering. If you're new to curry, start with 2 tablespoons; if you want more intense flavor, 3 tablespoons will do it.

Because the rice and chicken cook together, simply add a green salad to round out the meal.

For easy cleanup, cook in a baking dish that can go from stovetop to oven to table.

5 servings

Prep Time:
15 minutes or less

Total Time:
1 hour and 15 minutes or less

Nutritional Information
Per Serving (2 pieces of chicken)
Calories 695
Total Fat . . . . 33 g
Total Carbohydrate . . . . . . 57 g
Dietary Fiber . . . . 4 g
Sugars . . . . 12 g
Protein . . . . 42 g
Sodium . . . . 150 mg

Most supermarkets sell chicken cut into eight pieces. Cut the breast into four pieces for ten total pieces.

1 cut-up (3- to 4-pound) chicken, breast cut into 4 pieces
Salt and freshly ground black pepper
3 tablespoons vegetable oil
1 onion, chopped
2 garlic cloves, finely chopped
1½ cups basmati rice
2 to 3 tablespoons curry powder
1 teaspoon ground cumin
½ teaspoon ground ginger or 1 teaspoon finely chopped fresh ginger
½ teaspoon red pepper flakes, optional
3 cups reduced-sodium chicken broth
½ cup golden raisins or brown raisins
½ cup slivered almonds, lightly toasted

1. Preheat the oven to 350 degrees.

2. Sprinkle the chicken with salt and pepper.

3. In a large ovenproof skillet over medium-high heat, add the oil. Brown the chicken for 3 to 5 minutes per side. Remove the chicken and set aside. (You may need to brown the chicken in two or more batches, depending on the size of your skillet.)

4. Reduce the heat to medium and add the onion to the skillet. Sauté for 3 to 5 minutes, or until softened. Add the garlic and sauté for 1 minute. Add the rice, curry powder, cumin, ginger, and red pepper flakes and stir to combine. Add the broth and bring to a boil, scraping up any browned bits clinging to the pan. Return the chicken to the skillet and cover.

5. Bake for 30 to 40 minutes, or until the rice is tender, the broth has been absorbed, and the chicken is cooked through. Just before serving, add the raisins and almonds.

Tuna Salad

This colorful mayonnaise-based salad, served on a bed of greens, is full of healthful vegetables.

Add whichever embellishments you enjoy: olives, artichoke hearts, hard-boiled eggs, and cucumber are good options.

3 servings

Prep Time:
15 minutes or less

Total Time:
15 minutes or less

Nutritional Information
Per Serving (about ½ cup)
Calories 115
Total Fat . . . . 4 g
Total Carbohydrate . . . . 9 g
Dietary Fiber . . . . 3 g
Sugars . . . . 6 g
Protein . . . . 12 g
Sodium . . . . 220 mg

1 (5-ounce) can white tuna packed in water, drained
2 teaspoons regular or reduced-fat mayonnaise
½ teaspoon Dijon mustard
1 tablespoon finely chopped red onion
½ red, green, or yellow bell pepper, seeded and finely chopped
½ celery stalk, finely chopped
¼ cup matchstick carrots, finely chopped
Salt and freshly ground black pepper
6 cups mixed greens
2 tomatoes, cut into quarters (or eighths if large)

1. In a bowl, flake the tuna. Add the mayonnaise and mustard and stir to combine. Add the onion, bell pepper, celery, and carrots and stir gently to incorporate. Season with salt and pepper.

2. Divide the greens and tomatoes on three plates and top with a scoop of the tuna mixture.

Vegetarian Roll-Up

When you just want small bites, make a roll-up sandwich and slice off enough for a little meal. This way, you'll always have something ready to eat when you feel like it. Cover leftover slices with plastic wrap.

Adding an herbed or flavored cheese from the deli counter is a tasty way to add zing and calories. Choose any variety you like; Havarti with dill and Cheddar with horseradish are both good options. An herbed soft cheese spread, such as Boursin Garlic & Fine Herb, also can be used. For a blander taste, choose a plain cheese.

For added fiber and nutrition, sprinkle with extra veggies, such as shredded carrots.

1 serving

Prep Time:
15 minutes or less

Total Time:
15 minutes or less

**Nutritional Information
Per Serving**
Calories 490
Total Fat . . . . 30 g
Total Carbohydrate . . . . . . 37 g
Dietary Fiber . . . . 7 g
Sugars . . . . 4 g
Protein . . . . 18 g
Sodium . . . . 990 mg

2 large slices (about 2 ounces) Havarti with dill or plain Havarti cheese

1 (8-inch) whole wheat or plain flour tortilla or flatbread such as lavash

10 to 15 fresh spinach or arugula leaves

⅓ ripe avocado, chopped

⅓ cup roasted red peppers, patted dry and chopped

1. Place the cheese over the tortilla to cover. Microwave for 45 to 60 seconds on high. Layer the spinach, avocado, and red peppers on half of the tortilla. Roll up jellyroll style. Slice into 2-inch pieces.

Mulligatawny Soup

This curried chicken soup, richly flavored with apples, lemon, and cloves, was originally prepared by Indian cooks for British colonialists. They took the recipe back to England and later introduced it in the United States.

The interplay of flavors will have your tongue singing.

10 servings

Prep Time:
30 minutes or less

Total Time:
1 hour or less

Nutritional Information
Per Serving (about 1 cup)
Calories 145
Total Fat . . . . 4 g
Total Carbohydrate . . . . . . 15 g
Dietary Fiber . . . . 1 g
Sugars . . . . 4 g
Protein . . . . 12 g
Sodium . . . . 380 mg

2 tablespoons vegetable oil

1 carrot, chopped

1 onion, chopped

1 celery stalk, chopped

1 Granny Smith apple, peeled, cored, and chopped

2 tablespoons all-purpose flour

1 tablespoon curry powder

⅛ teaspoon ground cloves

6 cups reduced-sodium chicken broth

1 (14.5-ounce) can diced tomatoes, drained, or 1 ripe tomato, chopped

1 tablespoon fresh lemon juice

½ cup rice

1 pound boneless chicken breasts, cut into ¼-inch pieces

Salt and freshly ground black pepper

1. In a stockpot over medium-high heat, add the oil. Sauté the carrot, onion, celery, and apple for 8 to 10 minutes, or until softened. Add the flour, curry, and cloves and cook for 1 to 2 minutes, stirring constantly. Add the broth, tomatoes, and lemon juice and stir to combine. Bring to a boil. Add the rice and stir to combine. Reduce the heat, partially cover, and simmer for 10 minutes, stirring occasionally.

2. Add the chicken and cook for 5 to 10 minutes, or until the chicken and rice are cooked through. Season with salt and pepper.

Couscous with Almonds, Dried Blueberries, and Parmesan Cheese

This fast side dish is a multitextured combination of couscous, dried fruit, and crunchy almonds. Although a lot of people think that couscous is a grain, it is actually a type of semolina pasta.

Substitute golden raisins, brown raisins, dried cranberries, or chopped dried apricots for the dried blueberries if you prefer.

For stronger flavor, double the amount of garlic salt.

7 servings

Prep Time:
15 minutes or less

Total Time:
15 minutes or less

Nutritional Information
Per Serving
Calories 145
Total Fat . . . . 4 g
Total Carbohydrate . . . . . . 23 g
Dietary Fiber . . . . 2 g
Sugars . . . . 4 g
Protein . . . . 5 g
Sodium . . . . 200 mg

Lightly toasting the nuts gives them added flavor and crunch. Bake at 350 degrees for a few minutes, or cook in a dry skillet until golden and aromatic. Watch to make sure they don't burn.

1¼ cups reduced-sodium chicken broth
½ teaspoon garlic salt
1 cup couscous
1 tablespoon olive oil
¼ cup dried blueberries, golden raisins, or other small dried fruit
2 tablespoons grated or shredded Parmesan cheese, divided
2 tablespoons slivered almonds, lightly toasted

1. In a saucepan over medium-high heat, bring broth and garlic salt to a boil. Add the couscous, stir, cover, and remove from heat. Set aside for 5 minutes. Stir in oil, blueberries, and 1 tablespoon of the Parmesan cheese.

2. Just before serving, sprinkle with the remaining tablespoon of cheese and the almonds.

Adapted, with permission, from *Celebrate! Healthy Entertaining for Any Occasion* (Atlanta, GA: American Cancer Society, 2001), 194.

Honey-Teriyaki Salmon

This teriyaki topping is a great balance of sweet, savory, and salty and pairs perfectly with salmon, other fish, or chicken. With so many Asian condiments available at the market, it's easy to get a lot of flavor in one convenient ingredient, such as a teriyaki sauce. This recipe uses a teriyaki "glaze," which is thicker than the traditional sauce. Sold under various brand names (often called "Baste & Glaze"), the thicker glaze adds a more distinct coating. You can use any teriyaki sauce that is viscous; just avoid sauces with a thin, soy sauce–like consistency.

The secret of preparing fish is not to overcook it. The fish should be opaque on the inside, but still moist. Don't be afraid to poke and peek to make sure it's cooked through. Buy fillets that are the same thickness (about 1 inch) to ensure uniform cooking times.

Lining your pan with lightly oiled aluminum foil makes for easy cleanup. If you are sensitive to smells, this dish can also be cooked on an outdoor grill.

You can also use boneless, skinless chicken breasts in this dish. Because chicken breasts can be of varying thickness, pound them so they are more uniform for quicker and more even cooking. Chicken will take a couple of minutes longer than the fish to cook.

4 servings

Prep Time:
15 minutes or less

Total Time:
30 minutes or less

**Nutritional Information
Per Serving**
Calories 270
Total Fat . . . . 10 g
Total Carbohydrate . . . . . . 17 g
Dietary Fiber . . . . 0 g
Sugars . . . . 16 g
Protein . . . . 27 g
Sodium . . . . 1690 mg

If your doctor has advised that you follow a low-sodium diet or you are retaining fluid, this recipe may not be appropriate.

²/₃ **cup thick teriyaki sauce**

2 tablespoons honey

3 garlic cloves, finely chopped

1 (½-inch) piece fresh ginger, finely chopped

4 (4-ounce) 1-inch thick salmon fillets, patted dry

1. Place an oven rack in the upper middle position and pre-heat the oven to 500 degrees. Line a rimmed baking sheet with foil and lightly coat with nonstick cooking spray.

2. In a bowl, combine the teriyaki sauce, honey, garlic, and ginger. Reserve 2 tablespoons of the mixture.

3. Place the salmon fillets skin-side down on the baking sheet and lightly brush or spoon on the glaze.

4. Bake for 5 minutes. Remove from the oven and spread more glaze over the tops and sides of the salmon. Bake for an additional 5 minutes, or until the fish is cooked through.

5. Remove from the oven and brush with reserved glaze.

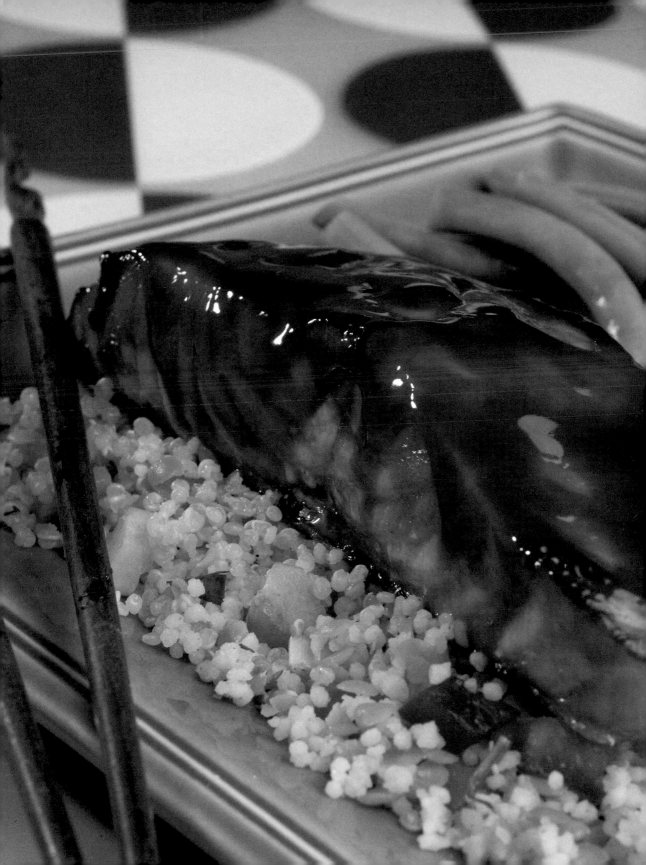

Southwest Bean Dip

This dip satisfies a craving for southwestern flavor but is still fine for a sensitive mouth. It has just enough chili powder to add spice without being too strong. Serve with soft tortillas or pita if your mouth is sensitive or carrot sticks and bell pepper strips for added fiber.

Garnish with fresh cilantro if you have some on hand.

Refrigerate for 30 minutes before serving for flavors to meld.

6 servings

Prep Time:
15 minutes or less

Total Time:
15 minutes or less

Nutritional Information
Per Serving (about ¼ cup)
Calories 95
Total Fat . . . . 5 g
Total Carbohydrate . . . . . . 10 g
Dietary Fiber . . . . 3 g
Sugars . . . . 0 g
Protein . . . . 4 g
Sodium . . . . 140 mg

Cannellini beans are also known as white kidney beans.

1 garlic clove
1 (15-ounce) can cannellini beans, rinsed and drained
Juice of 1 lime
2 tablespoons olive oil
1½ teaspoons chili powder
½ teaspoon ground cumin
¼ teaspoon salt

1. In a food processor, with the motor running, drop in the garlic and purée. Stop the machine, add the beans, half of the lime juice, the oil, chili powder, cumin, and salt, and process until smooth. Taste and add more lime juice, seasonings, or salt, if needed.

Spicy Cream of Broccoli Soup

This is a delicious way to eat healthful cruciferous vegetables and enjoy plenty of flavor in a low-fat, creamy soup.

Use caution when puréeing a hot soup. Cool slightly before puréeing, and avoid filling the blender or food processor more than three-quarters full.

5 servings

Prep Time:
15 minutes or less

Total Time:
30 minutes or less

Nutritional Information
Per Serving (about 1 cup)
Calories 115
Total Fat . . . . 4.5 g
Total Carbohydrate . . . . . . 13 g
Dietary Fiber . . . . 2 g
Sugars . . . . 9 g
Protein . . . . 7 g
Sodium . . . . 460 mg

The cayenne pepper and black pepper add heat, so carefully season to taste if experiencing mouth sores or omit for a mild soup.

To increase calories, substitute up to 1 cup heavy cream for an equal amount of milk.

This recipe may not be appropriate if you are experiencing gas.

3 cups broccoli florets and peeled stems, coarsely chopped
1½ cups reduced-sodium chicken broth, vegetable broth, or water
1 tablespoon olive oil
1 small (or ½ large) onion, finely chopped
1 tablespoon all-purpose flour
3 cups low-fat milk
½ teaspoon salt
½ teaspoon freshly ground black pepper
¼ teaspoon paprika
¼ teaspoon celery seed
Pinch cayenne pepper, or to taste, optional

1. In a large saucepan over high heat, bring the broccoli and broth to a boil. Reduce the heat, cover, and simmer for 8 to 10 minutes, or until very tender. Cool slightly. Transfer to a blender or food processor and purée. Set aside.

2. In the same saucepan over medium heat, add the oil. Sauté the onion for 3 to 5 minutes, or until softened. Add the flour and cook until fully incorporated, stirring constantly. Gradually add the milk and cook until thickened, stirring constantly. Add the reserved broccoli purée, salt, black pepper, paprika, celery seed, and cayenne pepper to the saucepan and stir well to combine.

Adapted, with permission, from *The American Cancer Society's Healthy Eating Cookbook, Third Edition* (Atlanta, GA: American Cancer Society, 2005), 41.

Chapter 6
UNINTENTIONAL WEIGHT LOSS

Unintentional weight loss can occur during cancer treatment. Some types of cancer and cancer treatment may increase your overall nutritional needs, including your need for calories. Maintaining your current weight can be challenging if you are experiencing side effects from treatment. Weight loss can increase fatigue, decrease muscular strength, affect your immune system, lengthen recovery, and decrease your overall quality of life.

If you are trying to prevent weight loss and maintain muscle mass, it is important to find ways to increase calories and protein in your diet. That often means supplementing a recipe you might otherwise make with extra protein or a higher-calorie alternative. The first recipe in this section, for example, is for Fortified Milk. This milk can be used in place of regular milk to add calories and protein to many dishes, and it is included as an ingredient in several shake recipes later in the chapter.

Many of the recipes in this section, like those found in other sections of the book, have small portion sizes. If you can eat often throughout the day, it will be easier to prevent weight loss.

Here are some suggestions to help you increase the amount of calories and protein in your diet:

- Consume 5 to 6 small meals or snacks a day, or try to eat every 2 to 3 hours. Nutritious snacks that are high in calories and/or protein include granola, trail mix, nuts, dried fruit, hard-boiled eggs, yogurt, peanut butter, cottage cheese, cheese, and canned chicken or tuna.

- Try smoothies, milkshakes, or canned nutritional supplements to add more calories, protein, and nutrients to your diet.

- If you get full quickly, drink the majority of your liquids between meals so that you are hungrier at meal times.

- Eat your favorite foods any time of day.

- Adding high-calorie foods such as sour cream, cream cheese, whipped cream, butter, and gravy to foods may be helpful in the short term to combat undesired weight loss.

Eat when you are hungriest—for many people, this is the morning. Don't be tied to conventions when it comes to what and when you eat. It's perfectly okay to have breakfast food for lunch or supper. Try combining foods that might not

N	Nausea
D	Diarrhea
C	Constipation
SM	Sore Mouth and Difficulty Swallowing
TA	Taste Alterations
WL	Unintentional Weight Loss

traditionally go together, such as in the Crunchy Peanut Butter Waffle Sandwich with Fresh Fruit on page 134. If you are trying to gain weight or prevent weight loss, take in as many healthful calories and as much protein as possible. Weight fluctuations are typical. You may lose weight the week after chemotherapy but gain most of it back before your next treatment. Discuss any large changes in weight with your medical team.

When weight loss is no longer a concern, resume a low-fat diet. A plant-based diet high in vegetables and fruit may help reduce the risk of cancer recurrence.

For more information about preventing weight loss,
contact the American Cancer Society at 800-227-2345
or visit our Web site at cancer.org.

Fortified Milk

Fortifying milk with nonfat instant dry milk adds protein and calories to your diet. Drink the milk by itself, add to a milkshake, or use in place of milk in your favorite recipe.

If the taste is too strong, dilute with liquid milk until palatable, or start with ¹/₂ cup of dry milk and gradually work up to 1 cup.

4 servings

Prep Time:
15 minutes or less

Total Time:
**15 minutes or less
plus 6 or more hours
refrigeration**

Nutritional Information
Per Serving (about 1 cup)
Calories 165
Total Fat . . . . 2.5 g
Total Carbohydrate . . . . . . 21 g
Dietary Fiber . . . . 0 g
Sugars . . . . 21 g
Protein . . . . 14 g
Sodium . . . . 200 mg

For added calories and calcium, substitute Fortified Milk for regular milk when making shakes, macaroni and cheese, puddings, and mashed potatoes.

1 quart low-fat milk
1 cup nonfat dry milk

1. In a container, blend low-fat milk and dry milk until dissolved. Cover and refrigerate for at least 6 hours.

Adapted, with permission, from *Nutrition for the Person with Cancer: A Guide for Patients and Families* [booklet] (Atlanta, GA: American Cancer Society, 2002), 16.

Peanut Butter Balls

This snack provides protein, calcium, and calories and is a yummy treat. For added texture, you can choose crunchy peanut butter or add chocolate chips or crispy rice cereal.

Adding dry milk provides extra calcium and protein. You won't even know it's there.

12 balls

Prep Time:
15 minutes or less

Total Time:
30 minutes or less

Nutritional Information
Per Serving (3 balls)
Calories 255
Total Fat . . . . 17 g
Total Carbohydrate . . . . . . 17 g
Dietary Fiber . . . . 2 g
Sugars . . . . 11 g
Protein . . . . 9 g
Sodium . . . . 25 mg

For added fiber and calories, add raisins or chopped dried apricots to the peanut butter mixture.

½ cup all-natural or regular creamy peanut butter
¼ cup instant dry milk
¼ cup confectioners sugar
¼ cup mini chocolate chips, optional
¼ cup crispy rice cereal, optional

1. In a bowl, combine the peanut butter, dry milk, and confectioners sugar and stir to incorporate. It will take a little time to mix the dry ingredients into the peanut butter. Add the chocolate chips and rice cereal and stir well to combine. Form the mixture into 1-inch balls and place on a plate. Cover and refrigerate for at least 20 minutes.

Super Protein Milkshake

For a high-protein, high-calorie drink, begin with Fortified Milk and enrich with ingredients such as Instant Breakfast, ice cream, and peanut butter.

2 servings

Prep Time:
15 minutes or less

Total Time:
15 minutes or less

**Nutritional Information
Per Serving (about 1 cup)**
Calories 295
Total Fat . . . . 6 g
Total Carbohydrate . . . . . . 51 g
Dietary Fiber . . . . 1 g
Sugars . . . . 41 g
Protein . . . . 11 g
Sodium . . . . 200 mg

1 cup Fortified Milk (see recipe, page 117)
½ cup ice cream
3 tablespoons chocolate or butterscotch syrup or malted milk powder
1 tablespoon creamy all-natural or regular peanut butter, optional
1 envelope Instant Breakfast mix

1. In a blender, combine the milk, ice cream, syrup, peanut butter, and Instant Breakfast and blend until smooth.

Add other ingredients from the same "flavor family" to intensify flavor. For example, pair chocolate or chocolate malt Instant Breakfast with chocolate ice cream and chocolate syrup or malted milk powder, or combine strawberry Instant Breakfast with strawberry ice cream. For milder flavors, start with vanilla Instant Breakfast or use vanilla ice cream.

Adapted, with permission, from *Eating Well, Staying Well During and After Cancer* (Atlanta, GA: American Cancer Society, 2004), 215.

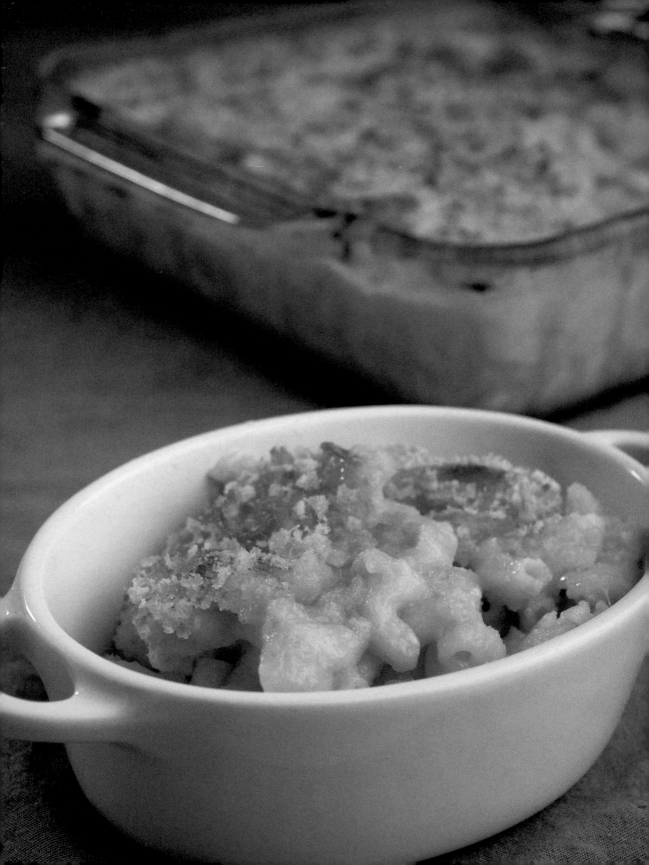

Creamy Mac and Cheese

When it comes to comfort food, nothing beats an ooey, gooey macaroni and cheese casserole. I first saw a version for this cooking method in an article by Julia Moskin in The New York Times and was dumbfounded. The pasta actually cooks in the sauce, making the prep time next to nothing. I streamlined the original recipe and added a breadcrumb topping for texture, and it's been a family favorite ever since.

For more authentic flavor, grate your own cheese (a shredder blade on a food processor is good for this) instead of buying packaged preshredded cheese.

8 servings

Prep Time:
15 minutes or less

Total Time:
1 hour and 15 minutes
or less

**Nutritional Information
Per Serving**
Calories 400
Total Fat . . . . 21 g
Total Carbohydrate . . . . . . 29 g
Dietary Fiber . . . . 1 g
Sugars . . . . 5 g
Protein . . . . 23 g
Sodium . . . . 510 mg

Try a combination of cheeses, using Gruyère for a nuttier flavor or Monterey Jack for a milder flavor. If you don't have any Parmesan cheese on hand, just leave it out.

Making homemade bread crumbs is a snap. Just throw a slice of bread in the food processor and process until it becomes crumbs.

2 cups low-fat milk
1 cup regular (not low-fat) cottage cheese
1 teaspoon dry mustard
Salt and freshly ground black pepper
1 pound sharp or extra-sharp Cheddar cheese, grated, divided
1 cup fresh bread crumbs
1 tablespoon grated Parmesan cheese, optional
½ pound uncooked elbow pasta

1. Preheat the oven to 375 degrees. Coat an 8-by-8-inch baking pan with nonstick cooking spray.

2. In a blender, combine the milk, cottage cheese, mustard, and a sprinkle of salt and pepper and blend until smooth.

3. In a bowl, combine 1 cup of the grated Cheddar cheese, the bread crumbs, and Parmesan cheese. Set aside.

4. In a large bowl, combine the remaining Cheddar cheese, the milk mixture, and uncooked pasta. Pour into prepared pan and cover tightly with foil.

5. Bake for 30 minutes. Uncover, stir gently, and top with reserved cheese mixture. Bake uncovered for an additional 20 minutes, or until just set. Let cool for 5 to 10 minutes before serving.

Egg Salad with Fresh Dill

Everyone has a favorite way to make hard-boiled eggs. One method to prevent the eggs from cracking during cooking is to place them in a saucepan and cover with an inch or two of cold water. Bring the water to a boil, cover the pan, remove from heat, and let stand for 12 minutes. Transfer the eggs to an ice-water bath and cool.

Serve the salad as a sandwich filling or with crisp lettuce and tomato wedges.

4 servings

Prep Time:
15 minutes or less

Total Time:
30 minutes or less

**Nutritional Information
Per Serving (about ½ cup)**
Calories 155
Total Fat . . . . 13 g
Total Carbohydrate . . . . 2 g
Dietary Fiber . . . . 0 g
Sugars . . . . 1 g
Protein . . . . 7 g
Sodium . . . . 190 mg

For stronger flavors,
add chopped capers,
crumbled blue cheese,
chopped tarragon or
other herbs, tomatoes,
or avocado.

3 tablespoons regular or reduced-fat mayonnaise

2 teaspoons Dijon mustard

4 hard-boiled eggs, coarsely chopped

2 teaspoons chopped fresh dill, optional

2 tablespoons finely chopped red onion, yellow onion, scallions, or chives

1 celery stalk, finely chopped

Salt and freshly ground black pepper

1. In a bowl, combine the mayonnaise and the mustard. Add the eggs, dill, onion, and celery and stir gently to incorporate. Season with salt and pepper.

Rosemary Beef with Shallot Cream Sauce

Tender lean beef, such as sirloin, is a good meat option and provides iron. The flavorful creamy sauce coats the meat without being too heavy.

Incorporating vegetables such as mushrooms and bell peppers into a skillet dish adds nutrients and flavor.

If your skillet is too small to cook all the ingredients at once, transfer the vegetables to a plate before adding the beef. To rewarm, return them to the pan just before the beef is finished cooking.

Serve this dish over rice or egg noodles if you wish.

4 servings

Prep Time:
15 minutes or less

Total Time:
30 minutes or less

Nutritional Information
Per Serving
Calories 280
Total Fat . . . . 16 g
Total Carbohydrate . . . . 7 g
Dietary Fiber . . . . 2 g
Sugars . . . . 3 g
Protein . . . . 26 g
Sodium . . . . 170 mg

2 tablespoons olive oil

2 shallots, finely chopped

1 red bell pepper, seeded and finely chopped

8 ounces mushrooms, sliced

1 pound lean steak, trimmed of excess fat, thinly sliced and cut into bite-sized pieces

1 teaspoon fresh rosemary, finely chopped

¼ teaspoon freshly ground black pepper

¼ teaspoon garlic salt

¼ cup regular or reduced-fat sour cream

2 tablespoons regular or reduced-fat cream cheese

1. In a large skillet over medium-high heat, add the oil. Sauté the shallots, red pepper, and mushrooms for 3 to 5 minutes, or until tender,

2. Sprinkle the steak with rosemary, pepper, and garlic salt. Add to the skillet and sauté for 3 to 5 minutes, or until lightly browned and just cooked through. Remove from heat and stir in the sour cream and cream cheese until smooth.

Adapted, with permission, from *Celebrate! Healthy Entertaining for Any Occasion* (Atlanta, GA: American Cancer Society, 2001), 216.

Mini Chicken Pot Pies

These miniature pies are sized for single servings. Keep extra cooked pies in the fridge to heat up for individual meals or freeze for later use. You will need four ramekins or oven-safe teacups for this recipe. To speed up the prep on the dish, roll out the crusts and start the filling while the chicken bakes.

4 pot pies

Prep Time:
30 minutes or less

Total Time:
**1 hour and 15 minutes
or less**

Nutritional Information
Per Serving (1 pot pie)
Calories 410
Total Fat . . . . 19 g
Total Carbohydrate . . . . . . 29 g
Dietary Fiber . . . . 2 g
Sugars . . . . 6 g
Protein . . . . 30 g
Sodium . . . . 470 mg

Frozen vegetables can be a huge timesaver and are as nutritious as fresh vegetables.

The chicken pot pie can also be baked in a larger dish for family-style eating. A round casserole dish should work. Bake for an additional 5 to 10 minutes, until the crust is golden.

---

1 pound boneless, skinless chicken breasts, halved
1 cup low-fat milk
2 tablespoons butter
1 small (or ½ large) onion, finely chopped
2 tablespoons all-purpose flour
1 cup reduced-sodium chicken broth
1 cup frozen peas and carrots mixture
Salt and freshly ground black pepper
1 refrigerated roll-out pie crust
1 egg combined with 1 tablespoon water, optional

1. Preheat the oven to 350 degrees.

2. In a baking pan, place the chicken in a single layer and add milk. Bake for 25 to 30 minutes, or until chicken is just cooked through. Remove the chicken and set aside to cool briefly, reserving the milk. Cut chicken into bite-sized pieces.

3. Increase the oven temperature to 425 degrees.

4. Meanwhile, in a large saucepan over medium heat, melt the butter. Sauté the onion for 3 to 5 minutes, or until softened. Add the flour and cook until fully incorporated, stirring constantly. Gradually add the broth and cook until thickened, stirring constantly. Add the reserved milk and cook until thickened. Add the peas and carrots and the chicken. Season with salt and pepper.

5. Divide chicken mixture evenly between four (1-cup) ramekins or oven-safe teacups. Roll out the crust and cut four circles; the circles should be big enough to overlap the edges of the ramekins by about 1 inch on all sides, but they need not be perfect circles. Top each ramekin with crust, pressing to seal the sides.

6. Brush the tops of the pies with the egg mixture. Cut a slit in the top of each crust. Place the ramekins on a baking sheet.

7. Bake for 12 to 18 minutes, or until the tops are golden. Let cool for 5 to 10 minutes before serving.

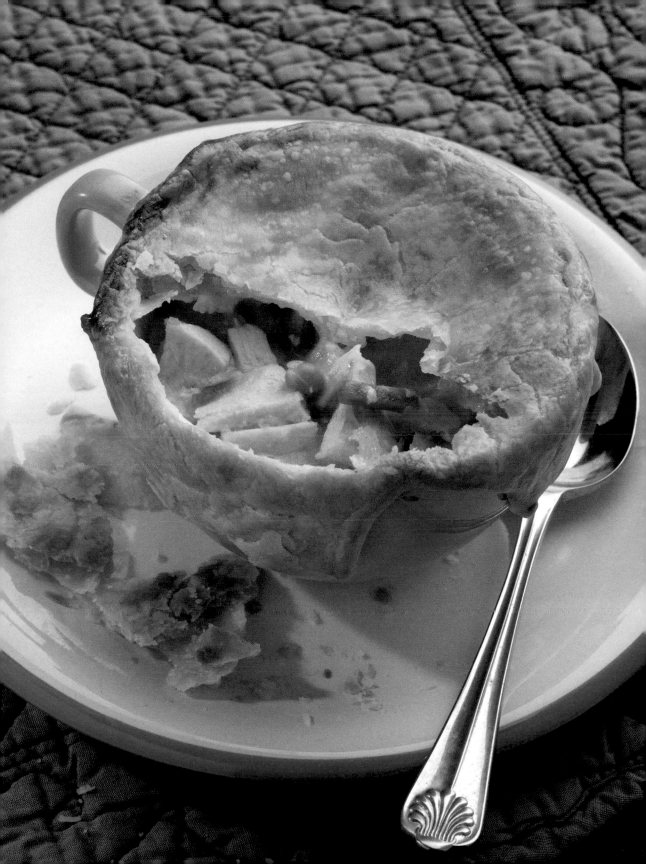

Classic Instant Breakfast Milkshake

Providing concentrated calories and nutrients, this rich drink is protein-packed. For variety, add strawberries, blueberries, peaches, bananas, or other fresh or frozen fruit.

Choose your favorite flavors of Instant Breakfast and ice cream. Increase flavor and calories by adding chocolate or strawberry syrup. You can also add peanut butter or dry milk for additional protein.

1 serving

Prep Time:
15 minutes or less

Total Time:
15 minutes or less

**Nutritional Information
Per Serving**
Calories 450
Total Fat . . . . 16 g
Total Carbohydrate . . . . . . 64 g
Dietary Fiber . . . . 1 g
Sugars . . . . 52 g
Protein . . . . 14 g
Sodium . . . . 260 mg

Despite its name, Instant Breakfast is a great way to add calories and protein any time of day. Look for the powdered version on the cereal aisle and mix with milk for a more economical alternative to canned nutritional supplements.

1 cup vanilla ice cream
½ cup low-fat milk or Fortified Milk (see recipe, page 117)
1 envelope Instant Breakfast mix

1. In a blender, combine the ice cream, milk, and Instant Breakfast and blend until smooth.

Adapted, with permission, from *Eating Well, Staying Well During and After Cancer* (Atlanta, GA: American Cancer Society, 2004), 212.

Cheese and Spinach Portobello Pizzas

Using a meaty portobello mushroom as the base of a "pizza" is good for those looking for a small vegetarian meal with nutritious ingredients.

For a slightly textured topping, use panko, Japanese bread crumbs. If your mouth is very sensitive, use store-bought or homemade soft bread crumbs, or omit the bread crumbs altogether and just top with cheese.

4 pizzas

Prep Time:
15 minutes or less

Total Time:
30 minutes or less

Nutritional Information
Per Serving (1 pizza)
Calories 180
Total Fat . . . . 10 g
Total Carbohydrate . . . . . . 13 g
Dietary Fiber . . . . 2 g
Sugars . . . . 7 g
Protein . . . . 10 g
Sodium . . . . 410 mg

Use the leftover ricotta cheese for Beef and Cheese Calzones (page 130).

4 large portobello mushroom caps, stems and gills removed, patted dry
2 teaspoons olive oil
³⁄₄ cup pasta sauce
¹⁄₂ cup shredded Italian blend or mozzarella cheese
¹⁄₄ cup regular or part-skim ricotta cheese
¹⁄₄ cup frozen chopped spinach, thawed, squeezed of excess liquid, and patted dry
Salt and freshly ground black pepper
¹⁄₄ cup panko or bread crumbs
2 tablespoons grated Parmesan cheese

1. Preheat the oven to 400 degrees. Line a rimmed baking sheet with foil and lightly coat with nonstick cooking spray.

2. Lightly brush the mushrooms with oil and place rounded side down on the baking sheet.

3. In a bowl, combine the pasta sauce, Italian blend cheese, ricotta cheese, and spinach. Season with salt and pepper. Divide the mixture among the four mushrooms and spread evenly.

4. In a separate bowl, combine the panko and Parmesan cheese. Sprinkle mixture on top of mushrooms.

5. Bake for 8 to 10 minutes, or until cheeses melt and mushrooms are heated through.

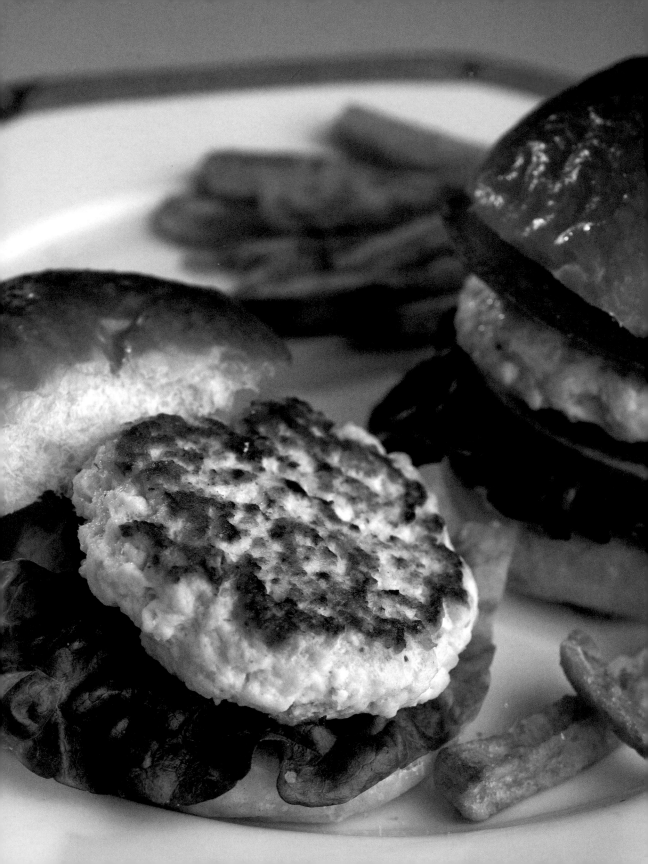

Mini Turkey Burgers

When you feel like a burger, but don't want a full-sized one, these "sliders" are just right. These mild-tasting burgers fit snugly in a small dinner roll or Hawaiian Sweet Roll to satisfy a craving without being too filling.

Choosing ground turkey breast makes sense if you are sensitive to the smell of beef or want a lower-fat option.

12 mini burgers

Prep Time:
30 minutes or less

Total Time:
30 minutes or less

**Nutritional Information
Per Serving (1 burger)**
Calories 180
Total Fat . . . . 4.5 g
Total Carbohydrate . . . . . . 20 g
Dietary Fiber . . . . 1 g
Sugars . . . . 2 g
Protein . . . . 14 g
Sodium . . . . 250 mg

Top burgers with a dollop of ketchup or cranberry relish (page 95) and serve with sweet potato fries.

Add cheese for extra calories and protein.

1 egg
1 pound ground turkey breast
2 tablespoons finely chopped onion or 1 shallot, finely chopped
2 tablespoons plain bread crumbs
2 tablespoons regular or reduced-fat sour cream
1 tablespoon Dijon mustard
1 tablespoon vegetable oil
12 (2½-inch) dinner rolls

1. In a bowl, beat the egg. Add the turkey, onion, bread crumbs, sour cream, and mustard. Form the mixture into twelve (2-inch) patties.

2. In a large skillet over medium-high heat, add the oil. Cook the burgers for 4 to 6 minutes per side, or until golden and cooked through. To ensure the inside is cooked through, cover the skillet for the last 1 to 2 minutes of cooking.

Beef and Cheese Calzones

Calzones, stuffed pizzas, are easy to prepare by using store-bought refrigerated pizza dough. Refrigerated pizza dough is softer and puffier than most restaurant doughs, which makes it better for people with sensitive mouths.

The choice of fillings is limited only by your imagination. Just resist the temptation to overstuff. You can also make your own pizza dough or buy it at many supermarket bakery departments.

4 calzones

Prep Time:
15 minutes or less

Total Time:
30 minutes or less

**Nutritional Information
Per Serving (1 calzone)**
Calories 515
Total Fat . . . . 19 g
Total Carbohydrate . . . . . . 56 g
Dietary Fiber . . . . 2 g
Sugars . . . . 12 g
Protein . . . . 31 g
Sodium . . . . 1340 mg

Use leftover ricotta cheese for Cheese and Spinach Portobello Pizzas (page 127).

½ pound extra-lean ground beef (preferably 93 percent lean)
1 small onion, finely chopped, optional
1¼ cups shredded Italian blend or mozzarella cheese, divided
1 cup pasta sauce, plus extra for dipping
2 tablespoons regular or part-skim ricotta cheese, optional
1 (13.8-ounce) can refrigerated pizza dough
1 teaspoon olive oil
4 teaspoons grated Parmesan cheese

1. Preheat the oven to 425 degrees.

2. In a skillet over medium-high heat, cook the beef and onion for 6 to 8 minutes, or until the meat is no longer pink and the onion softens, stirring frequently to break up the meat. Drain if needed. Transfer to a bowl and add 1 cup of the Italian blend cheese, pasta sauce, and ricotta cheese, and stir gently to combine. Set aside.

3. Unroll dough on a lightly oiled 10-by-15-inch baking sheet. Starting at the center, press out dough with your hands to form a 14-by-8-inch rectangle. Cut into four 7-by-4-inch rectangles and separate slightly.

4. Sprinkle 1 tablespoon of the Italian blend cheese on half of each rectangle, to within 1 inch of the crusts' edges. Divide beef mixture evenly on top of the cheese. Fold the dough over filling. Press edges securely and pinch to seal. Prick tops with fork. Separate calzones slightly if needed. Brush lightly with oil and sprinkle each calzone with 1 teaspoon of the Parmesan cheese.

5. Bake for 12 to 16 minutes, or until golden brown.

Peach Yogurt Frost

This frosty, mild drink is an easy snack or mini meal. Replacing ice cubes with frozen peaches or other frozen fruit adds flavor.

Choose a fruit combination that appeals to you. For example, make a strawberry shake by substituting frozen strawberries, strawberry yogurt, and strawberry-flavored mix.

3 servings

Prep Time:
15 minutes or less

Total Time:
15 minutes or less

Nutritional Information
Per Serving (about ¾ cup)
Calories 155
Total Fat . . . . 1.5 g
Total Carbohydrate . . . . . . 30 g
Dietary Fiber . . . . 1 g
Sugars . . . . 24 g
Protein . . . . 7 g
Sodium . . . . 95 mg

1 cup low-fat milk or Fortified Milk (see recipe, page 117)
1 cup frozen peaches or 6 to 10 crushed ice cubes
1 (6-ounce) container peach low-fat yogurt
1 envelope vanilla Instant Breakfast mix

1. In a blender, combine the milk, peaches, yogurt, and Instant Breakfast and blend until smooth.

Adapted, with permission, from *Eating Well, Staying Well During and After Cancer* (Atlanta, GA: American Cancer Society, 2004), 212.

Peanut Noodles

These peanut noodles get an Asian spin from flavorful soy sauce, sesame oil, and fresh ginger. If you prefer a hotter, spicier dish, add a drop or two of chili oil or a pinch of red pepper flakes.

4 servings

Prep Time:
30 minutes or less

Total Time:
30 minutes or less

Nutritional Information
Per Serving
Calories 280
Total Fat . . . . 16 g
Total Carbohydrate . . . . . . 26 g
Dietary Fiber . . . . 2 g
Sugars . . . . 3 g
Protein . . . . 8 g
Sodium . . . . 290 mg

For added flavor and texture, top with chopped peanuts or julienned snow peas, bell peppers, or cucumber.

4 ounces linguine, spaghetti, or soba noodles
¼ cup creamy all-natural or regular peanut butter
2 tablespoons reduced-sodium soy sauce
2 tablespoons Asian sesame oil
1 tablespoon red wine vinegar or rice wine vinegar
1 tablespoon chopped fresh ginger
1 garlic clove, chopped
1 teaspoon honey, optional

1. Prepare the pasta according to package directions. After draining, rinse with cold water.

2. Meanwhile, in a blender, combine the peanut butter, soy sauce, sesame oil, vinegar, ginger, garlic, and honey and blend until smooth.

3. In a bowl, combine the sauce and drained pasta and stir gently to incorporate. If the sauce is too thick, dilute with hot water, 1 tablespoon at a time.

Mediterranean Pita Pocket

A warm pita bread sandwich filled with a creamy dip and crumbled soft cheese is a welcome small meal. For added flavor, mix fresh mint and olives into the hummus.

1 serving

Prep Time:
15 minutes or less

Total Time:
15 minutes or less

Nutritional Information
Per Serving
Calories 280
Total Fat . . . . 15 g
Total Carbohydrate . . . . . . 28 g
Dietary Fiber . . . . 5 g
Sugars . . . . 4 g
Protein . . . . 11 g
Sodium . . . . 840 mg

2 tablespoons hummus (see recipe, page 53, or use store-bought)
2 tablespoons crumbled feta cheese
1 tablespoon chopped fresh mint, optional
4 kalamata olives, pitted and chopped
½ whole wheat or plain pita
2 to 3 thin slices tomato
4 to 5 thin slices cucumber

1. In a bowl, combine the hummus, feta, mint, and olives.

2. Microwave the pita on high for 10 seconds, or until just warm. Fill with hummus mixture and line with tomato and cucumber slices.

Crunchy Peanut Butter Waffle Sandwich with Fresh Fruit

Choose your favorite fruits to nestle in this newfangled sandwich. Sliced bananas or straw-berries are always good, but in the fall you can also try apples or pears. If you are out of fresh fruit, substitute jam.

Not a peanut butter fan? Plain or fruit-flavored cream cheese also makes a tasty filling.

1 serving

Prep Time:
15 minutes or less

Total Time:
15 minutes or less

Nutritional Information
Per Serving
Calories 660
Total Fat . . . . 40 g
Total Carbohydrate . . . . . . 59 g
Dietary Fiber . . . . 7 g
Sugars . . . . 25 g
Protein . . . . 18 g
Sodium . . . . 400 mg

2 multigrain or other frozen waffles
3 tablespoons all-natural or regular peanut butter
1 tablespoon honey
6 to 8 slices strawberry or ripe banana

1. Toast waffles according to package directions and let cool briefly. Spread one waffle with peanut butter and drizzle with honey. Evenly distribute fruit slices and top with the remaining waffle.

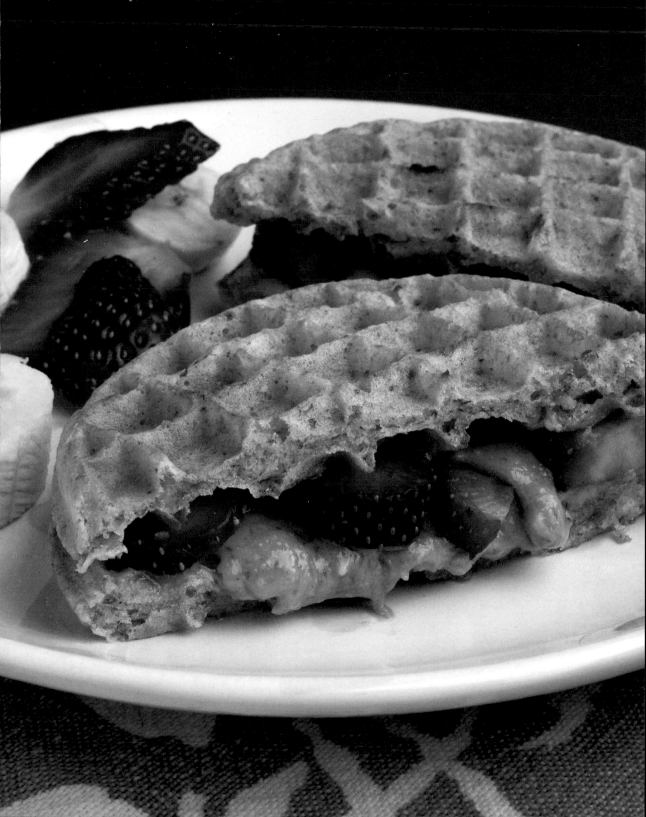

Fruity Chicken Salad

Each bite of this salad provides a burst of flavor and texture from the mixture of chicken, dried sweetened cranberries, crunchy apples, and toasted almonds.

If you want to avoid mayonnaise, substitute a vinaigrette or Italian dressing. For something a little sweeter, substitute vanilla yogurt.

While not essential, adding fresh herbs gives the salad vibrancy. If you have some in your fridge or garden, snip a few leaves.

4 servings

Prep Time:
15 minutes or less

Total Time:
15 minutes or less

Nutritional Information
Per Serving (about 1 cup)
Calories 245
Total Fat . . . . 13 g
Total Carbohydrate . . . . . . 14 g
Dietary Fiber . . . . 3 g
Sugars . . . . 10 g
Protein . . . . 18 g
Sodium . . . . 100 mg

Toasting nuts brings out their flavor and adds crunch. Bake at 350 degrees for about 5 minutes or cook in a dry skillet until golden and aromatic. Cool before using.

2 cups (about 8 ounces) chopped cooked chicken
2 scallions, thinly sliced
1 apple, chopped
1 celery stalk, finely chopped
¼ cup dried sweetened cranberries
2 to 3 tablespoons regular or reduced-fat mayonnaise
2 tablespoons chopped fresh basil or Italian parsley or 1 tablespoon chopped fresh tarragon, optional
Salt and freshly ground black pepper
¼ cup slivered almonds, lightly toasted

1. In a bowl, combine the chicken, scallions, apple, celery, cranberries, and 2 tablespoons of the mayonnaise. Add the herbs and stir gently to incorporate. Add more mayonnaise if necessary. Season with salt and pepper. Add the toasted almonds just before serving. If you're not eating all of the salad at once, add the nuts to individual servings right before eating to keep them crunchy.

Grilled Peanut Butter–Banana–Chocolate Panini

Elvis should be smiling down on this sandwich. Nutella, a creamy chocolate and hazelnut spread, is a perfect replacement for the chocolate chips in this sandwich. Just spread the peanut butter on one piece of bread, Nutella on the other, and sandwich the banana slices between them before grilling.

If you have a panini press, use it for making this sandwich. If not, just press the sandwich down with a spatula. If possible, cut 1-inch slices from a hearty loaf of bakery-style white bread to use in this sandwich—the thicker bread will hold up better during cooking.

1 serving

Prep Time:
15 minutes or less

Total Time:
15 minutes or less

**Nutritional Information
Per Serving**
Calories 710
Total Fat . . . . 34 g
Total Carbohydrate . . . . . . 87 g
Dietary Fiber . . . . 7 g
Sugars . . . . 22 g
Protein . . . . 19 g
Sodium . . . . 590 mg

This sandwich blends sweet and savory while providing calories and nutrients.

If bananas are unappealing, swirl raspberry jam or your favorite fruit spread into the peanut butter.

2 tablespoons all-natural or regular peanut butter

2 tablespoons mini chocolate chips, 2 ounces finely chopped chocolate, or 2 tablespoons Nutella or other chocolate spread

2 (1-inch thick) slices sturdy white bread, egg bread, or other sliced bread

½ small ripe banana, thinly sliced

1 teaspoon butter, softened

1. In a bowl, combine the peanut butter and mini chocolate chips. Spread on one side of each piece of bread. Place banana on top of one slice of bread and top with the other slice, peanut butter side down. Spread the butter on the other sides of the bread. Place in a panini press or skillet over medium heat.

2. Cook until both sides are golden and the chocolate has melted, turning carefully and firmly pressing the top of the sandwich with a spatula if you are using a skillet.

The Survival Kit

Good nutrition and adequate caloric intake can help you maintain energy, stamina, and strength during your treatment. Unfortunately, many types of treatment affect your appetite and desire to eat. Take advantage of times when you feel hungry, since the feeling may not last long.

Consider making a "survival kit" to keep handy next to your favorite chair, spot on the couch, or your bed. There may be times when you feel like eating, but don't feel like going to the kitchen or asking someone to prepare a snack for you. Keep an insulated lunch box or small cooler close by with some quick and easy snacks or drinks to capitalize on moments when you want to eat. Supplies kept close at hand can help you maintain your weight and hydration when your appetite is poor.

Here are some suggestions for your cooler:

- Make sure to have beverages on hand, such as water, juice boxes, and sports drinks. Canned nutritional supplements can help when you feel like drinking but not eating.

- Use an ice pack for keeping foods cold, such as yogurt, individually wrapped cheeses, cottage cheese, hard-boiled eggs, gelatin, puddings, and sandwiches.

- Crackers, pretzels, applesauce, and single-serving canned fruits may be easier to digest if you are feeling nauseated.

- Granola bars, trail mix, peanut butter, sandwiches, and dips with beans or cheese can add variety and protein to your snacks.

- Try to keep a mixture of sweet and salty snacks on hand to satisfy any cravings you might have.

- Single-serving and resealable packaging are helpful and prevent waste if your appetite is poor.

Kitchen Staples

Cancer and its treatment can cause changes in your eating habits and your appetite. Your appetite may fluctuate, and your tastes may change frequently. A well-stocked pantry can help you quickly prepare a healthy meal or snack.

Cupboard and Countertop

Canned beans, such as black beans, chickpeas, cannellini beans, pinto beans, kidney beans, black-eyed peas, and refried beans (not cooked in lard)

Grains, such as white rice, brown rice, quinoa, wheatberries, bulgur, barley, and packaged precooked rice

Pastas (whole wheat or white) such as penne, bowties, macaroni, orzo, couscous, egg noodles, soba, and ramen noodles

Pretzels, whole wheat or regular crackers, breadsticks, dry cereals, granola, vanilla wafers, graham crackers, animal crackers, and popcorn

Hot cereals, such as oatmeal (quick-cooking and rolled oats) and Cream of Wheat

Flour, cornmeal, bread crumbs, and pancake mix

Onions, potatoes, garlic

Canned tomatoes (diced or whole), tomato sauce, salsa, pizza and pasta sauces, and ketchup

Canned fruits in juice, such as fruit cocktail, pears, mandarin oranges, and peaches

Canned pumpkin purée

Applesauce

Tomatoes

Bananas

Dried fruits, such as raisins, sweetened cranberries, apricots, prunes, and blueberries

Canned soups and broths

Canned meats, such as tuna, salmon, and chicken

Peanut butter (all-natural or regular), Nutella

Pudding and flavored gelatin

Nuts, such as almonds (whole and slivered), walnuts, and sunflower seeds

Flavored drink mixes, Instant Breakfast, and nonfat dry milk

Decaffeinated tea bags

Evaporated milk (regular or skim)

Vinegars, such as red wine, white, and balsamic

Oils, including olive oil, canola oil, and nonfat cooking spray

Honey, light brown sugar, white sugar, and confectioners sugar

Refrigerator

Vegetables and fruits

Reduced-fat milk and buttermilk or lactose-free milk and kefir

Reduced-fat or regular plain and flavored yogurt (without added sugar) and Greek yogurt

Reduced-fat or regular cheeses, such as Cheddar, mozzarella, feta, Monterey Jack, Parmesan, string cheese, and cottage cheese

Reduced-fat or regular sour cream and cream cheese

Flour or corn tortillas

Eggs

Minced garlic

Sauces, such as Worcestershire, soy, teriyaki, and chili

Salad dressing and condiments, Dijon mustard

Other beverages, such as sports drinks, 100 percent fruit and vegetable juices, and liquid supplements

Precooked mashed potatoes

Hummus

Freezer

Frozen vegetables, fruits, and canned juice concentrates (100 percent juices)

Frozen chopped onions and chopped green pepper

Breads, such as whole grain breads, dinner rolls, English muffins, bagels, pita bread, and bobolis

Lean meats, such as chicken breast, ground turkey breast, and extra-lean ground beef

Fish, such as salmon, flounder, tilapia, and red snapper

Frozen desserts, such as frozen yogurt, fruit sorbet, ice cream, sherbet, and Popsicles

Frozen waffles

Tips for Dining Out

Eating out occasionally is one way to increase your intake of calories and protein. People tend to eat more in social settings. When eating out you also have more food choices and, in most restaurants, you will be well removed from any cooking aromas that might bother you or disturb your appetite.

- Try to dine early to avoid crowds. Wait staff may be more accommodating to special requests during meal times that are less busy.

- Consider telling your server that you are undergoing cancer treatment and that your tastes and appetite have been affected. Ask if the restaurant will provide small portions. Perhaps they have half-portions or lunch portions that are smaller than a normal entrée.

- Ask if you can order from the children's or senior citizen's menu.

- Ask if you can taste small amounts of certain foods before ordering to see whether they will work for you.

- Ask if you can order à la carte and choose side dishes only.

- Ask if you can split a meal with someone else for no extra charge.

Avoiding Excess Weight Gain During Treatment

Not every chemotherapy regimen produces side effects that make it difficult to eat. Some patients may gain weight during treatment. Weight gain may be due to decreased physical activity, hormonal changes, consuming more comfort foods, consuming more calories overall, or eating more frequently. Below are suggestions to help prevent unwanted weight gain.

Ask your oncologist if you can exercise during treatment. If so, try some type of physical activity most days of the week. Any physical activity you enjoy is good. For example, start walking 5 to 10 minutes a day and work up to at least 30 minutes a day at a moderate pace. A moderate pace means that you are still able to talk while walking briskly. Other ideas include dancing, biking, yoga, and pilates.

Limit the sugar and sweet foods you eat. These foods contribute calories without necessary nutrients.

Limit your overall fat intake. Replace saturated fat with healthier fats such as nuts and seeds (for example, walnuts and pumpkin seeds), olive oil and canola oil, and fatty fish (such as salmon, mackerel, tuna, and sardines).

Increase the amount of fiber in your diet. Fiber will help you feel full and maintain regularity. High-fiber foods include vegetables and fruit with the peel or skin left on, whole grains (brown rice, whole wheat pasta, cereal, and whole wheat bread), nuts, and beans or peas.

Decrease your portion sizes, especially of foods high in calories, fat, and added sugars.

Do not skip meals, and try to eat your largest meal early in the day. It is okay to have snacks as long as they are healthy and you don't eat more overall.

Pay attention to what triggers you to eat, and think about whether you are eating for reasons other than hunger. Some people eat because of stress, boredom, in response to television ads, or to meet an emotional need.

While aggressive weight loss is not recommended during treatment, a modest amount of weight loss (1 to 2 pounds per week) during treatment is generally acceptable as long as your oncologist approves, your weight loss is monitored, and your weight loss does not interfere with treatment.

Resource List

American Cancer Society
Toll-free: 800-227-2345
Web site: http://www.cancer.org

The American Cancer Society (ACS) is the nationwide community-based volunteer health organization dedicated to eliminating cancer as a major health problem by preventing cancer, saving lives, and diminishing suffering from cancer, through research, education, advocacy, and service. For comprehensive, up-to-date cancer information, visit the Web site or call the National Cancer Information Center, toll-free, 24 hours a day, 7 days a week. The American Cancer Society offers a wide variety of educational programs, services, and referrals, as well as information related to nutrition during cancer treatment.

The American Cancer Society does not necessarily endorse the agencies, organizations, corporations, and publications represented in this resource guide. This guide is provided for assistance in obtaining information only.

Organizations Providing Health, Food, Diet, and Supplement Information

American Dietetic Association (ADA)
120 South Riverside Plaza, Suite 2000
Chicago, IL 60606-6995
Toll-free: 800-877-1600
Web site: http://www.eatright.org

The ADA is the world's largest organization of food and nutrition professionals. The ADA serves the public by promoting nutrition, health, and well-being. The Web site contains information on diet and nutrition, publications, and a registered dietitian locator service, including access to dietitians who specialize in oncology nutrition.

International Food Information Council (IFIC) Foundation
1100 Connecticut Avenue, NW
Suite 430
Washington, DC 20036
Phone: 202-296-6540
Fax: 202-296-6547
Web site: http://ific.org

As the educational arm of the IFIC, the IFIC Foundation communicates science-based information on food safety and nutrition to health and nutrition professionals, educators, journalists, and others for distribution to consumers. The IFIC has established partnerships with a wide range of professional organizations and academic institutions to develop science-based information for the public.

Meals on Wheels Association of America (MOWAA)
203 S. Union Street
Alexandria, VA 22314
Telephone: 703-548-5558
Fax: 703-548-8024
Web site: http://www.mowaa.org
E-mail: mowaa@mowaa.org

Meals on Wheels is a membership association of programs that provide home-delivered and group meals. The goal of the organization is to improve the quality of life of the needy, particularly the elderly, disabled, and homebound. Some programs may provide other health and social services such as transportation, recreation, nutrition, education, information, referrals, and case management.

Memorial Sloan-Kettering Cancer Center (MSKCC)
About Herbs, Botanicals, and Other Products
http://www.mskcc.org/mskcc/html/11570.cfm

Memorial Sloan-Kettering Cancer Center's About Herbs, Botanicals, and Other Products Web site provides information for consumers about herbs, botanicals, and alternative or unproven cancer therapies, including details about adverse effects, interactions, and potential benefits or problems.

Office of Dietary Supplements (ODS)
National Institutes of Health
6100 Executive Boulevard
Room 3B01, MSC 7517
Bethesda, Maryland 20892-7517
Phone: 301-435-2920
Fax: 301-480-1845
Web site: http://ods.od.nih.gov
E-mail: ods@nih.gov

The ODS supports research and shares research results about dietary supplements. To explore the role of dietary supplements in the improvement of health care, the ODS plans, organizes, and supports conferences, workshops, and symposia on scientific topics related to dietary supplements.

Quackwatch
Web site: http://www.quackwatch.com

Quackwatch is a nonprofit corporation whose purpose is to combat health-related frauds, myths, fads, and fallacies.

United States Department of Agriculture (USDA)
1400 Independence Avenue, SW
Washington, DC 20250
Telephone: 202-720-2791
Web site: http://www.usda.gov
E-mail: AgSec@usda.gov

The USDA strives to enhance the quality of life for the American people by supporting production of agriculture. The USDA is also responsible for the food supply, managing agricultural products, forests, and rangeland, and community development.

USDA Food and Nutrition Information Center (FNIC)
National Agricultural Library
10301 Baltimore Avenue, Room 105
Beltsville, MD 20705
Telephone: 301-504-5414
Fax: 301-504-6409
Web site: http://www.nal.usda.gov/fnic

The USDA's FNIC is an information center for the National Agricultural Library. FNIC materials and services include dietitians and nutritionists available to answer inquiries, publications on food and nutrition, and resource lists and bibliographies. The FNIC Web site includes information on dietary supplements, food safety, dietary guidelines, food composition facts (including fast food), a list of available publications, and information on popular topics.

United States Food and Drug Administration (FDA)
5600 Fishers Lane
Rockville, MD 20857
Toll-free: 888-INFO-FDA (888-463-6332)
Fax: 301-443-9767
Web site: http://www.fda.gov

The FDA is an agency within the U.S. Department of Health and Human Services and consists of eight centers/offices. The FDA is a public health agency charged with protecting Americans by enforcing the Federal Food, Drug, and Cosmetic Act and other laws, promoting health by helping safe and effective products reach the market in a timely manner, and monitoring products for continued safety after they are in use. The FDA regulates food, cosmetics, medicines, biologics, medical devices, and radiation-emitting consumer products, as well as feed and drugs for pets and farm animals. The Web site has extensive information about all the products the FDA regulates.

Center for Food Safety and Applied Nutrition (CFSAN) Outreach and Information Center
5100 Paint Branch Parkway (HFS-555)
College Park, MD 20740-3835
Toll-free: 888-SAFEFOOD (888-723-3366)
TYY: 800-877-8339
Web site: http://www.cfsan.fda.gov

The goal of the Outreach and Information Center is to enhance CFSAN's ability to provide and respond to the public's desire and demand for more useful, timely, and accurate information regarding its regulated products. In addition to providing food safety information, the Outreach and Information Center provides assistance with other CFSAN issues, including nutrition, dietary supplements, food labeling, cosmetics, food additives, and food biotechnology.

United States Pharmacopeia (USP)
12601 Twinbrook Parkway
Rockville, MD 20852-1790
Toll-free: 800-227-8772
Telephone: 301-881-0666
Web site: http://www.usp.org/

The USP is dedicated to producing quality control standards for the strength, quality, and purity of pharmaceuticals. In 1997, the USP began publishing standards for dietary supplements. These standards focus on the strength, quality, purity, packaging, and labeling of dietary supplements and are updated yearly.

Organizations Providing Health and Cancer Information

Centers for Disease Control and Prevention (CDC)
1600 Clifton Road NE
Atlanta, GA 30333
Toll-free: 800-CDC-INFO (800-232-4636)
TTY: 888-232-6348
Web site: http://www.cdc.gov
E-mail: cdcinfo@cdc.gov

The CDC is an agency of the U.S. Department of Health and Human Services. Their mission is to promote health and quality of life by preventing and controlling disease, injury, and disability. Their Web site contains a searchable map of the 12 centers, offices, and institutes, information about health topics, downloadable publications, and links to related sources.

National Cancer Institute (NCI)
NCI Public Inquiries Office
6116 Executive Boulevard, Room 3036A
Bethesda, MD 20892-8322
Toll-free: 800-4-CANCER (800-422-6237)
TTY: 800-332-8615
Web site: http://www.cancer.gov

This government agency, as part of the National Institutes of Health, provides information on cancer research, diagnosis, and treatment through several services. People with cancer, caregivers, and health care professionals may call the NCI's toll-free telephone service for cancer-related information. Includes information about complementary and alternative medicine and nutrition in cancer care. Spanish-speaking staff and Spanish materials are available.

Cancer Information Service (CIS)
Toll-free: 800-4-CANCER (800-422-6237)
TTY: 800-332-8615
Web site: http://cis.nci.nih.gov

The CIS provides information to consumers and health care professionals. The Web site contains a wealth of information, including pamphlets and brochures on cancer diagnosis, treatment, research, and prevention. Spanish-speaking staff is available.

Office of Cancer Complementary and Alternative Medicine (OCCAM)
National Cancer Institute (NIH)
6116 Executive Boulevard
Suite 609, MSC 8339
Bethesda, MD 20892
Toll-free: 800-4-CANCER (800-422-6237)
Telephone: 301-435-7980
Fax: 301-480-0075
Web site: http://www.cancer.gov/CAM
E-mail: ncioccam1-r@mail.gov

The OCCAM coordinates and enhances the activities of the NCI in the arena of complementary and alternative medicine. The goal of the OCCAM is to increase the amount of high-quality cancer research and information about the use of complementary and alternative modalities.

National Library of Medicine (NLM)
8600 Rockville Pike
Bethesda, MD 20894
Telephone: 301-402-1384
Fax: 301-594-5983
Web site: http://www.nlm.nih.gov
E-mail: custserv@nlm.nih.gov

The NLM collects, organizes, and makes available biomedical science information to investigators, educators, and practitioners and carries out programs designed to strengthen medical library services in the United States. Its electronic databases are used extensively throughout the world by both health professionals and the public. Materials are available in languages other than English.

MEDLINEplus
Web site: http://medlineplus.gov

MEDLINEplus is a database for consumer health information, including dictionaries; articles and journals from other organizations; textbooks, newsletters, and health news for online reading; and links to organizations that provide consumer information and clearinghouses that send health literature.

NLM Gateway
Web site:
http://gateway.nlm.nih.gov/gw/Cmd

The NLM Gateway offers links to searchable databases and allows users to search simultaneously in multiple retrieval systems.

PubMed
Web site:
http://www.ncbi.nlm.nih.gov/PubMed

This database provides access to millions of literature references and abstracts in MEDLINE and other databases, with links to on-line journals. The site is searchable by keyword.

Index

About the Authors

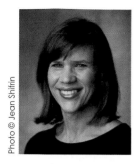

Jeanne Besser, formerly a syndicated food columnist and stylist for the *Atlanta Journal-Constitution*, has been a food writer for more than 15 years. *What to Eat During Cancer Treatment* is her fifth cookbook. Her other cookbooks include *The First Book of Baking* (1996), *Working Mom's Fast and Easy One-Pot Cooking* (1998, revised as *Working Mom's Fast & Easy Family Cookbook* in 2003), *The 5:30 Challenge: 5 Ingredients, 30 Minutes, Dinner on the Table* (2006), and *The Great American Eat-Right Cookbook* (2007). Jeanne resides in Montclair, New Jersey.

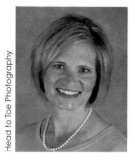

Kristina (Kris) Ratley, RD, CSO, LDN, is a registered dietitian and works as a dietitian on call with the South Atlantic Division of the American Cancer Society. Kris is a Board Certified Specialist in Oncology Nutrition with more than 20 years of experience in the field of dietetics. Her personal accomplishments include completing three marathons, and she hopes to run in the New York City Marathon soon. Kris lives in North Myrtle Beach, South Carolina.

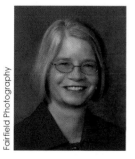

Sheri Knecht, RD, CSO, CNSD, LDN, is a registered dietitian and manager of the Dietitian on Call program for the South Atlantic Division of the American Cancer Society. She founded the Dietitian on Call program in 2000 and works within that program to promote good nutrition and physical activity for cancer patients and survivors. Sheri is a Board Certified Specialist in Oncology Nutrition and a Certified Nutrition Support Dietitian. She resides in Norfolk, Virginia.

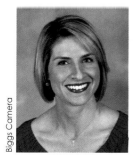

Michele Szafranski, MS, RD, CSO, LDN, is a registered dietitian and works as a dietitian on call with the South Atlantic Division of the American Cancer Society. Michele is a Board Certified Specialist in Oncology Nutrition. She lives in Charlotte, North Carolina.

Books Published by
the American Cancer Society

Available everywhere books are sold and online at **cancer.org/bookstore**

General Cancer Information
The American Cancer Society: A History of Saving Lives
The Cancer Atlas (available in English, Spanish, French, Chinese)
Cancer: What Causes It, What Doesn't
The Tobacco Atlas, Third Edition (available in English, Spanish, French, Chinese)

Information for People with Cancer
American Cancer Society's Complete Guide to Colorectal Cancer
Breast Cancer Clear & Simple: All Your Questions Answered
QuickFACTS™ Advanced Cancer
QuickFACTS™ Bone Metastasis
QuickFACTS™ Colorectal Cancer, Second Edition
QuickFACTS™ Lung Cancer
QuickFACTS™ Thyroid Cancer

Emotional Support
Chemo and Me: My Hair-Loss Experience (illustrated)
Get Better! Communication Cards for Kids & Adults (bilingual communication cards)
The Survivorship Net: A Parable for the Family, Friends, and Caregivers of People with Cancer
What Helped Get Me Through: Cancer Survivors Share Wisdom and Hope

Coping with Symptoms and Side Effects
American Cancer Society's Guide to Pain Control, Revised Edition
Lymphedema: Understanding and Managing Lymphedema After Cancer Treatment

Support for Families and Caregivers
Cancer Caregiving A to Z: An At-Home Guide for Patients and Families
Cancer in the Family: Helping Children Cope with a Parent's Illness
Couples Confronting Cancer: Keeping Your Relationship Strong
When the Focus Is on Care: Palliative Care and Cancer

Books for Children
Because…Someone I Love Has Cancer: Kids' Activity Book (5 twist-up crayons included)
Healthy Me: A Read-Along Coloring & Activity Book
Jacob Has Cancer: His Friends Want to Help (coloring book)
Kids' First Cookbook: Delicious-Nutritious Treats to Make Yourself!
Let My Colors Out
Mom and the Polka-Dot Boo-Boo
Nana, What's Cancer?
No Thanks, but I'd Love to Dance
Our Dad Is Getting Better
Our Mom Has Cancer (available in hard cover and paperback)
Our Mom Is Getting Better

Tools for the Health Conscious
*American Cancer Society Complete Guide to Nutrition for Cancer Survivors:
    Eating well, Staying Well During and After Cancer Treatment, Second Edition*
American Cancer Society's Healthy Eating Cookbook, Third Edition
Celebrate! Healthy Entertaining for Any Occasion
The Great American Eat-Right Cookbook
Kicking Butts: Quit Smoking and Take Charge of Your Health, Second Edition
National Health Education Standards: Achieving Excellence, Second Edition
Reduce Your Cancer Risk

Inspirational Survivor Stories
Angels & Monsters: A child's eye view of cancer
Crossing Divides: A Couple's Story of Cancer, Hope, and Hiking Montana's Continental Divide
I Can Survive (illustrated)